Advances in Heart Electrotherapy

Advances in Heart Electrotherapy

Editors

Ewa Lewicka
Alicja Dąbrowska-Kugacka
Aleksandra Liżewska-Springer

MDPI • Basel • Beijing • Wuhan • Barcelona • Belgrade • Manchester • Tokyo • Cluj • Tianjin

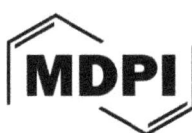

Editors
Ewa Lewicka
Department of Cardiology
and Electrotherapy
Medical University of Gdansk
Gdansk
Poland

Alicja Dąbrowska-Kugacka
Department of Cardiology
and Electrotherapy
Medical University of Gdansk
Gdansk
Poland

Aleksandra
Liżewska-Springer
Department of Cardiology
and Electrotherapy
Medical University of Gdansk
Gdansk
Poland

Editorial Office
MDPI
St. Alban-Anlage 66
4052 Basel, Switzerland

This is a reprint of articles from the Special Issue published online in the open access journal *International Journal of Environmental Research and Public Health* (ISSN 1660-4601) (available at: www.mdpi.com/journal/ijerph/special_issues/Heart_Electrotherapy).

For citation purposes, cite each article independently as indicated on the article page online and as indicated below:

LastName, A.A.; LastName, B.B.; LastName, C.C. Article Title. *Journal Name* **Year**, *Volume Number*, Page Range.

ISBN 978-3-0365-6571-2 (Hbk)
ISBN 978-3-0365-6570-5 (PDF)

© 2023 by the authors. Articles in this book are Open Access and distributed under the Creative Commons Attribution (CC BY) license, which allows users to download, copy and build upon published articles, as long as the author and publisher are properly credited, which ensures maximum dissemination and a wider impact of our publications.
The book as a whole is distributed by MDPI under the terms and conditions of the Creative Commons license CC BY-NC-ND.

Contents

About the Editors vii

Preface to "Advances in Heart Electrotherapy" ix

Paul-Mihai Boarescu, Iulia Diana Popa, Cătălin Aurelian Trifan, Adela Nicoleta Roşian and Ştefan Horia Roşian
Practical Approaches to Transvenous Lead Extraction Procedures—Clinical Case Series
Reprinted from: *Int. J. Environ. Res. Public Health* **2022**, *20*, 379, doi:10.3390/ijerph20010379 . . . 1

Jedrzej Michalik, Alicja Dabrowska-Kugacka, Katarzyna Kosmalska, Roman Moroz, Adrian Kot and Ewa Lewicka et al.
Hemodynamic Effects of Permanent His Bundle Pacing Compared to Right Ventricular Pacing Assessed by Two-Dimensional Speckle-Tracking Echocardiography
Reprinted from: *Int. J. Environ. Res. Public Health* **2021**, *18*, 11721, doi:10.3390/ijerph182111721 . 17

Aleksandra Liżewska-Springer, Tomasz Królak, Karolina Dorniak, Maciej Kempa, Alicja Dabrowska-Kugacka and Grzegorz Sławiński et al.
Right Ventricular Endocardial Mapping and a Potential Arrhythmogenic Substrate in Cardiac Amyloidosis—Role of ICD
Reprinted from: *Int. J. Environ. Res. Public Health* **2021**, *18*, 11631, doi:10.3390/ijerph182111631 . 27

Łukasz Tułecki, Anna Polewczyk, Wojciech Jacheć, Dorota Nowosielecka, Konrad Tomków and Paweł Stefańczyk et al.
A Study of Major and Minor Complications of 1500 Transvenous Lead Extraction Procedures Performed with Optimal Safety at Two High-Volume Referral Centers
Reprinted from: *Int. J. Environ. Res. Public Health* **2021**, *18*, 10416, doi:10.3390/ijerph181910416 . 33

Marek Czajkowski, Wojciech Jacheć, Anna Polewczyk, Jarosław Kosior, Dorota Nowosielecka and Łukasz Tułecki et al.
The Influence of Lead-Related Venous Obstruction on the Complexity and Outcomes of Transvenous Lead Extraction
Reprinted from: *Int. J. Environ. Res. Public Health* **2021**, *18*, 9634, doi:10.3390/ijerph18189634 . . . 47

Zofia Lasocka, Alicja Dabrowska-Kugacka, Ewa Lewicka, Aleksandra Liżewska-Springer and Tomasz Królak
Successful Catheter Ablation of the "R on T" Ventricular Fibrillation
Reprinted from: *Int. J. Environ. Res. Public Health* **2021**, *18*, 9587, doi:10.3390/ijerph18189587 . . . 63

Łukasz Tułecki, Anna Polewczyk, Wojciech Jacheć, Dorota Nowosielecka, Konrad Tomków and Paweł Stefańczyk et al.
Analysis of Risk Factors for Major Complications of 1500 Transvenous Lead Extraction Procedures with Especial Attention to Tricuspid Valve Damage
Reprinted from: *Int. J. Environ. Res. Public Health* **2021**, *18*, 9100, doi:10.3390/ijerph18179100 . . . 69

Maciej Kempa, Andrzej Przybylski, Szymon Budrejko, Tomasz Fabiszak, Michał Lewandowski and Krzysztof Kaczmarek et al.
Utilization of Subcutaneous Cardioverter-Defibrillator in Poland and Europe–Comparison of the Results of Multi-Center Registries
Reprinted from: *Int. J. Environ. Res. Public Health* **2021**, *18*, 7178, doi:10.3390/ijerph18137178 . . . 83

Dorota Nowosielecka, Wojciech Jacheć, Anna Polewczyk, Łukasz Tułecki, Andrzej Kleinrok and Andrzej Kutarski
Prognostic Value of Preoperative Echocardiographic Findings in Patients Undergoing Transvenous Lead Extraction
Reprinted from: *Int. J. Environ. Res. Public Health* **2021**, *18*, 1862, doi:10.3390/ijerph18041862 . . . **91**

Michał Orszulak, Artur Filipecki, Wojciech Wróbel, Adrianna Berger-Kucza, Witold Orszulak and Dagmara Urbańczyk-Swić et al.
Regional Strain Pattern Index—A Novel Technique to Predict CRT Response
Reprinted from: *Int. J. Environ. Res. Public Health* **2021**, *18*, 926, doi:10.3390/ijerph18030926 . . . **111**

About the Editors

Ewa Lewicka

Prof. Ewa Lewicka is a scientific researcher and academic teacher in the Department of Cardiology and Heart Electrotherapy at the Medical University of Gdańsk, Poland. For many years, she has been interested in cardiac electrotherapy and treatment using permanent cardiac pacing, ICD and the ablation methods. She is the author or co-author of many papers on this subject in peer-reviewed journals. Her research interests also include pulmonary hypertension, diagnosis and treatment of pulmonary arterial hypertension and CTEPH. Currently, she is the chair-elect of the Pulmonary Circulation Section of the Polish Cardiac Society. Since 2018, she has been the head of the Cardio-Oncology Outpatient Clinic in Gdańsk and organizes an annual conference on this subject (Baltic Cardio-Oncology Conference). She is currently conducting research projects in the field of cardio-oncology.

Alicja Dąbrowska-Kugacka

Alicja Dąbrowska-Kugacka completed a degree in Medicine at the Medical University of Gdańsk in Poland in 1991 and at the University of Antwerpen in Belgium in 1992. In 1997, she completed her PhD thesis, and in 2013, the habilitation entitled: "Haemodynamics of cardiac contraction during various types of atrial pacing". She is a specialist in internal medicine and cardiology. She has been working as a staff cardiologist at the Department of Cardiology and Electrotherapy, Medical University of Gdansk, since 1992. She is a university teacher for 30 years, experienced in clinical and laboratory research, chairman and lecturer of national and international medical conferences, and author of more than 140 publications in international journals with impact factor. Her major interests include general cardiology, but specially electrotherapy, cardiac pacing, cardiac resynchronization therapy, echocardiography, pulmonary hypertension, cardiomyopathies, heart failure, atrial fibrillation and sport medicine.

Aleksandra Liżewska-Springer

Aleksandra Liżewska-Springer completed her medical studies at the University of Gdańsk (Poland), including a semester at the University of Turku in Finland. In 2019, she defended her PhD thesis regarding echocardiographic assessment of hemodynamics in patients undergoing pulmonary vein isolation.

Currently, she is undergoing cardiology residency at the Department of Cardiology and Electrotherapy of the University Clinical Centre in Gdańsk (Poland). Her interests include arrhythmias, cardiomyopathies including cardiac amyloidosis, cardio-oncology, echocardiography and ultrasonography.

Preface to "Advances in Heart Electrotherapy"

The introduction of permanent cardiac pacing in the late 1950s began the era of cardiac electrotherapy. In the 1980s, implantable cardioverter defibrillators (ICDs) were introduced. These advances created new challenges for cardiac implantable electronic devices (CIEDs). Right ventricular pacing was the primary breakthrough; however, over the years, it has become apparent that it can induce cardiac contraction dyssynchrony. Biventricular pacing allowed for the alleviation of dyssynchrony and improved the survival of patients with heart failure and bundle branch block. In recent decades, His bundle pacing has become a new strategy for physiological ventricular activation. However, the use of CIEDs carries several risks, e.g., complications related to transvenous leads. This led to the development of percutaneous lead extraction techniques as well as the introduction of a subcutaneous ICD (S-ICD) and leadless pacing. Technological evolution promises an exciting future in the development of cardiac electrotherapy.

In this Special Issue, readers can find out about the clinical and hemodynamic aspects of right ventricular, His bundle, and biventricular pacing; ICD therapy; treatment of complications and technological advances in cardiac electrotherapy.

Ewa Lewicka, Alicja Dąbrowska-Kugacka, and Aleksandra Liżewska-Springer
Editors

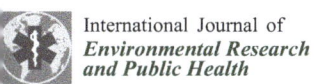

Case Report

Practical Approaches to Transvenous Lead Extraction Procedures—Clinical Case Series

Paul-Mihai Boarescu [1,2], Iulia Diana Popa [2], Cătălin Aurelian Trifan [2,3], Adela Nicoleta Roșian [2,*] and Ștefan Horia Roșian [2,4,*]

1. Department of Pharmacology, Toxicology and Clinical Pharmacology, Iuliu Hațieganu University of Medicine and Pharmacy Cluj-Napoca, Gheorghe Marinescu Street, No. 23, 400337 Cluj-Napoca, Romania
2. "Niculae Stăncioiu" Heart Institute Cluj-Napoca, Calea Moților Street, No. 19-21, 400001 Cluj-Napoca, Romania
3. Department of Cardiovascular Surgery, "Iuliu Hațieganu" University of Medicine and Pharmacy Cluj-Napoca, 19-21 Calea Moților Street, 400001 Cluj-Napoca, Romania
4. Department of Cardiology—Heart Institute, "Iuliu Hațieganu" University of Medicine and Pharmacy Cluj-Napoca, 19-21 Calea Moților Street, 400001 Cluj-Napoca, Romania
* Correspondence: adelarosianu@gmail.com (A.N.R.); dr.rosianu@gmail.com (Ș.H.R.); Tel.: +40-745-071-333 (A.N.R.); +40-744-337-227 (Ș.H.R.)

Abstract: Transvenous lead extraction (TLE) is regarded as the first-line strategy for the management of complications associated with cardiac implantable electronic devices (CIEDs), when lead removal is mandatory. The decision to perform a lead extraction should take into consideration not only the strength of the clinical indication for the procedure but also many other factors such as risks versus benefits, extractor and team experience, and even patient preference. TLE is a procedure with a possible high risk of complications. In this paper, we present three clinical cases of patients who presented different indications of TLE and explain how the procedures were successfully performed. In the first clinical case, TLE was necessary because of device extravasation and suspicion of CIED pocket infection. In the second clinical case, TLE was necessary because occlusion of the left subclavian vein was found when an upgrade to cardiac resynchronization therapy was performed. In the last clinical case, TLE was necessary in order to remove magnetic resonance (MR) non-conditional leads, so the patient could undergo an MRI examination for the management of a brain tumor.

Keywords: transvenous lead extraction; cardiac implantable electronic devices; clinical cases

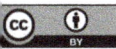

1. Introduction

As more people have been living longer in recent decades, the use of cardiac implantable electronic devices (CIEDs) has increased significantly. CIEDs include permanent pacemakers (PPMs) and implantable cardioverter-defibrillators (ICDs). Since the beginning of the 21st century, there has been an expansion of the indications for CIEDs. Even more, device therapy has become more complex, frequently involving multiple leads per patient and more sophisticated devices [1].

Lead removal is currently a specialized procedure with well-defined indications, as patients' longer life expectancy has led to an increase in the number of device-related complications and, consequently, to an increased need to perform lead-removal procedures [2].

Transvenous lead extraction (TLE) is regarded as the first-line strategy for the management of complications associated with CIEDs when lead removal is mandatory [3]. Minor complications of TLE, which include bleeding, pocket hematoma, pneumothorax, venous thrombosis, and migrated lead fragments, even if they are usually not life-threatening, are significant and require rapid intervention [4]. Pericardial tamponade is the most common major complication. Other major complications include hemothorax, thromboembolic events, vascular laceration, cardiac avulsion, and even death. Some of the considerable

TLE complications may entail emergent sternotomy and surgical repair, and, in rare cases of rapid and massive blood loss, death is often the outcome [4]. The rate of the major complications that require emergent intervention were reported to be low (up to 2.2% of cases) [5,6], while the mortality rate was reported to be exceedingly low (0.3%) [7]. Male gender, age during TLE, higher NYHA class, low left ventricle ejection fraction, presence of atrial fibrillation, and chronic renal failure were identified as the main factors predicting shorter survival among patients undergoing TLE [8].

The present study aims to highlight the indications and the methods of transvenous lead extraction and to present some clinical cases where lead extraction was mandatory and procedures were successfully performed without major or minor complications.

2. Clinical Cases

All the procedures were performed in the electrophysiology room, with patients in deep analgesia-sedation and monitored by an anesthesiologist. Moreover, a cardio-thoracic surgeon and a cardiovascular surgery operating room were on stand-by in the same building.

2.1. First Clinical Case

2.1.1. Patient's Medical History and Presentation

A 54-year-old male with a history of a chronically implanted ICD (at another center in a foreign country) was initially admitted to the Cardiology Department because of pocket erosion and possible pocket infection, as shown in Figure 1.

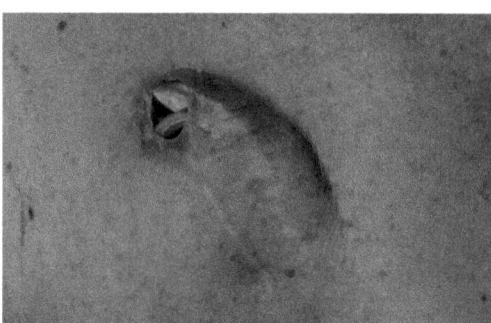

Figure 1. The aspect of the pocket erosion with the extravasation of the device and the lead, at the moment of admission to the hospital.

The medical history of the patient revealed that he has three-vessel coronary artery disease and that his first ICD, with a passive fixation double-coil lead, was implanted 11 years before this admission, as the primary prevention of sudden cardiac death. After three years, due to inappropriate internal electric shocks, a diagnosis of lead fracture was established. A new dual-coil active fixation lead was implanted, and the ICD generator was replaced without extraction of the old lead. Due to battery discharge, the ICD generator was replaced again one year later.

At the time of admission to our department, the patient was asymptomatic. The ECG showed a sinus rhythm with left bundle-branch block. A chest X-ray revealed an increased cardiothoracic ratio, a pulse-generator ICD placed subcutaneously in the left subclavian area, and two dual-coil defibrillation leads in the apex of the right ventricle (Figure 2).

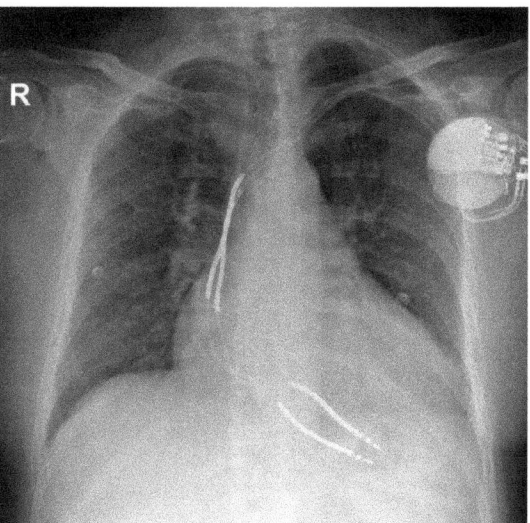

Figure 2. Chest X-ray at the time of admission at the hospital.

The transthoracic echocardiogram revealed a markedly dilated left ventricle, severe reduction in global contractility (EF: 21%), a restrictive filling pattern, moderate mitral regurgitation, and moderate tricuspid regurgitation without visualization of vegetations. A transesophageal echocardiography was also performed, and no intracavitary vegetation was identified at the tricuspid valve or leads' level.

Biochemical evaluation excluded systemic inflammation, as C reactive protein, fibrinogen, and the erythrocytes sedimentation rate were all in normal ranges. The blood cultures and wound-drainage cultures were also negative.

2.1.2. Transvenous Leads Extraction Procedure

The ICD pulse generator was interrogated using a corresponding programmer, which revealed repeated episodes of fast ventricular tachycardia (VT), interpreted as ventricular fibrillation (VF), with adequate internal electric shock administration. The last episode was recorded 10 months ago. Before starting the procedure, the anti-tachycardia therapies were discontinued. CIED fluoroscopy was performed to identify the position of the ICD pulse generator in the left subclavian area. One double coil, with an active fixation ICD lead (dwell time 8 years), was connected to the pulse generator and tracked normally. Another double coil, with a passive fixation ICD lead (dwell time 11 years), was noted to be fractured, with the proximal end lead remnant in the ICD pocket. Iodinated contrast media was injected into the peripheral vein of the left arm, without revealing subclavian or brachiocephalic vein occlusion.

After deep analgesia-sedation, an incision was made, and the pulse generator was removed from the pocket. Afterward, the leads were dissected to the level of the anchoring sleeves, to free them up from the scar tissue. The lead connected to the ICD pulse generator was disconnected, the tie-down sutures were removed, and gentle traction was initiated to remove the lead, without success. The connector of the lead was cut off and a Liberator locking stylet was advanced and locked at the tip of the lead. The Liberator locking stylet was secured on the lead using a one-tie accessory. With continuous traction, a 13 French bidirectional, rotational, mechanical lead-extraction sheath (Evolution RL, Cook Medical, USA) was advanced over the lead, up to its tip, to break up the heavy fibrosis from the left innominate vein, lateral wall of the left atrium, proximal pole of the lead, and lead's tip. After removing the fibrosis, continuous gentle traction dislodged the lead, and it was completely removed without difficulty (as shown in Supplementary Video S1).

A similar technique was used for the abandoned lead, and the same 13 French bidirectional rotational mechanical lead extraction sheath was used and advanced over the lead, up to its tip, to break up the heavy fibrosis near the superior vena cava, lateral wall of the left atrium, tricuspid valve, the proximal pole of the lead, and lead's tip. After removing the heavy fibrosis, continuous gentle traction dislodged the lead, and it was completely removed without incident (as shown in Supplementary Video S2).

The overall fluoroscopy time for this procedure was 4 min and 13 s.

The extracted leads with extensive fibrosis, especially on the coils of the leads, are shown in Figure 3.

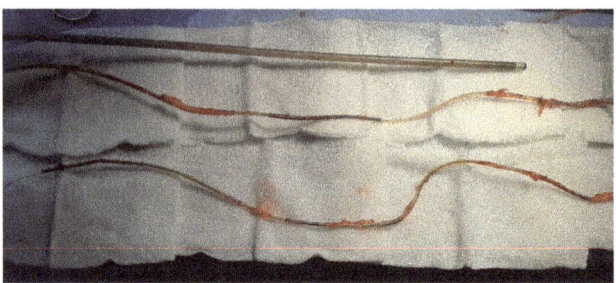

Figure 3. Extracted leads with extensive fibrosis.

A transthoracic echocardiogram was performed immediately after the procedure in the electrophysiology room. No pericardial effusion tricuspid valve dysfunction, or lead fragments were found. Subsequently, the patient was monitored (also by echocardiography) for 24 h in the intensive care unit for critical cardiac patients.

After 16 days of antibiotic therapy with Vancomycin, a new ICD was implanted on the right side of the chest (Figure 4).

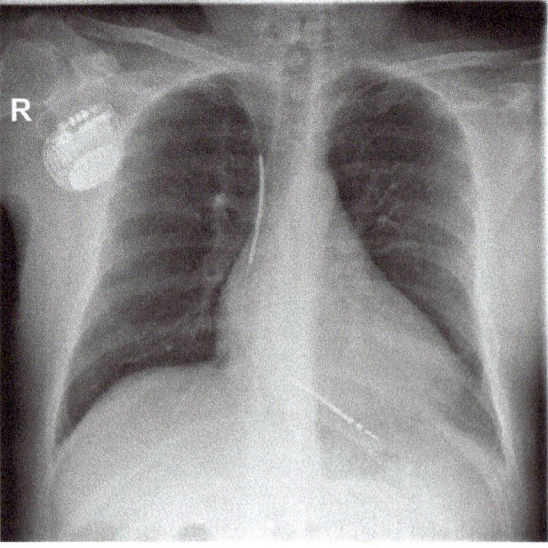

Figure 4. Chest X-ray with new defibrillator on the right side of the chest and the lead implanted through the right subclavian vein.

2.2. Second Clinical Case

2.2.1. Patient's Medical History and Presentation

A 67-year-old male patient with a dual-chamber pacemaker was admitted to the Cardiology Department for an upgrade to his cardiac resynchronization therapy due to impaired systolic function. The patient was diagnosed with ischemic cardiomyopathy, chronic heart failure (HF) with III New York Heart Association (NYHA) functional status, and a dual-chamber pacemaker for third-degree atrioventricular block had been implanted seven years before the current admission to the hospital.

At the time of admission to our department, the patient complained of considerable limitations to physical activity due to shortness of breath and fatigue despite optimal medical therapy. An ECG showed an atrial sinus rhythm with a ventricular-paced rhythm. A chest X-ray revealed an increased cardiothoracic ratio, a pulse generator PM placed subcutaneously in the left subclavian area, and two bipolar active fixation leads—one in the right atrial appendage and the other on the apex of the right ventricle.

The echocardiogram revealed a mildly dilated left ventricle, a severe reduction in global contractility (EF: 23%), a restrictive filling pattern, mild aortic regurgitation, moderate mitral regurgitation, moderate tricuspid regurgitation, diffuse hypokinesia, and no visible vegetations.

A pacemaker interrogation revealed 100% atrial sensed, 100% ventricular paced, and no underlying rhythm, with both leads having impedance, pacing, and sensing parameters within normal limits.

2.2.2. Transvenous Leads Extraction Procedure

The first intention was to implant only the left ventricular lead (LV) in a branch of the coronary sinus (CS), maintaining the pre-existing RA and RV leads for an upgrade to a CRT-P, although, according to current guidelines [9], the indication was that a CRT-D would provide the patient maximum benefits.

Iodinated contrast media was injected into the peripheral vein of the left arm, revealing occlusion of the left subclavian vein, with collateral circulation developed in the chest and neck and the suspicion of minimal circulation present on the deep subclavian venous axis (as shown in Figure 5).

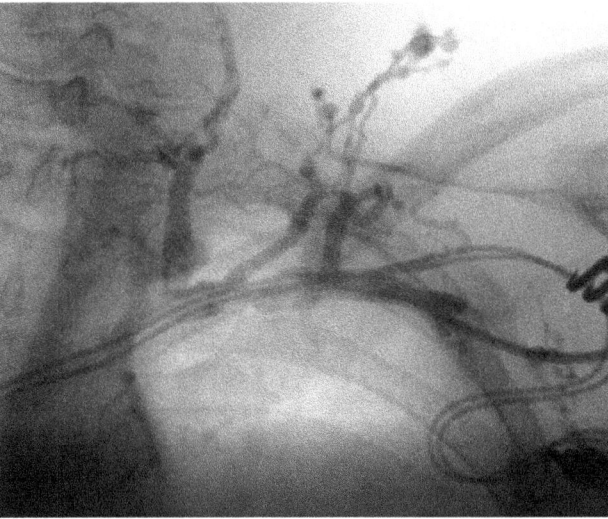

Figure 5. Occlusion of the left subclavian vein, with collateral circulation.

Axillary vein puncture was performed, and a J-tip guidewire was advanced only up to the subclavian vein, indicating possible occlusion at this level. An Abbott 0.014″ hydrophilic guide was introduced to identify the remaining lumen. The hydrophilic guide also stopped at this level, demonstrating the impossibility of passage on the deep venous axis due to occlusion.

As the patient was pacemaker-dependent, temporary cardiac pacing was performed using the right femoral vein approach, maintaining a stand-by heart rate of 50 beats/min, and hemodynamically monitoring was assured.

After deep analgesia-sedation, an incision was made, and the pulse generator was extracted. The two leads were disconnected and dissected up to the sutures at the level of the cephalic vein, to release them from the scar tissue. Tie-down sutures were removed, and gentle traction was made to easily mobilize the two leads, without the possibility of withdrawing them.

At that time, it was decided to extract the RV (dwell time 7 years) lead, being the only possibility to reach into the heart and to replace it with a single-coil defibrillation lead.

The same technique described in Case 1 was used: a Liberator locking stylet was advanced up to the top of the lead, locked at this level, and secured using a one-tie accessory. The right atrium (RA) lead was secured with a guidewire. With continuous traction, a 9 French bidirectional, rotational, mechanical lead-extraction sheath (Evolution RL, Cook Medical, Bloomington, IN, USA) was advanced with difficulty over the lead, up to the left brachiocephalic vein, without the possibility of going further (as shown in Supplementary Video S3). Under these circumstances, the sheath was withdrawn, revealing large deposits of fibrin on the tip of the sheath. A new 11 French bidirectional, rotational, mechanical lead-extraction sheath (Evolution RL, Cook Medical, USA) was used and advanced over the lead up to the RA level. At this level, the RV lead detached from the RV apex was easily extracted (as shown in Supplementary Video S4).

The extracted lead with the large deposits of fibrin removed from the tip of the 9 French bidirectional, rotational, mechanical lead-extraction sheath can be seen in Figure 6.

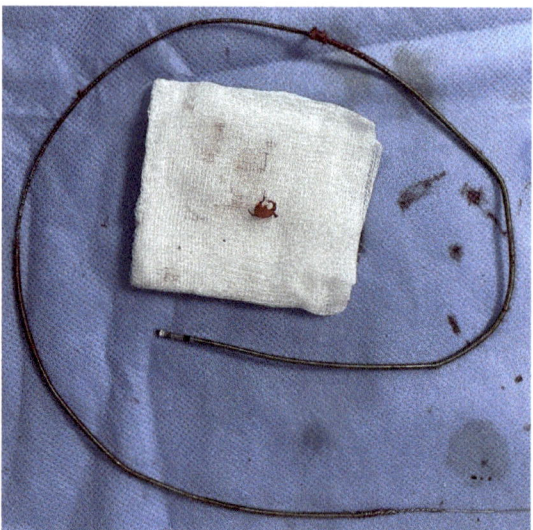

Figure 6. Extracted ventricular lead with large deposits of fibrin.

The outer sheath of the Evolution RL system was kept at the RA level. Two 0.035″/180 cm J-tip guidewires were inserted in the RA through this sheath. Afterward, the RA lead was checked, proving to have impedance, pacing, and sensing parameters within normal limits, which demonstrated that it was functional and could be preserved.

One of the 0.035″/180 cm J-tip guidewires was used to introduce a Biotronik Selectra Bio 2 45 cm sheath (Biotronik, Berlin, Germany), and a single-coil, DF-4 active fixation defibrillation lead was inserted in the apical RV apex through this sheath. On the other remaining 0.035″/180 cm J-tip guidewire, a Biotronik Selectra "Multipurpose EP (MPEP)" 55 cm sheath was used to cannulate the coronary sinus. After standard occlusive coronary sinus venography was performed, a suitable posterolateral vein was identified, and an IS4, OTW lead, was placed on that vein. After revision of the pre-pectoral pocket, the three leads were connected to a CRT-D.

The overall fluoroscopy time for this procedure was 15 min.

Post-procedural echocardiography revealed no pericardial effusion, no additional tricuspid valve dysfunction, and no lead fragments. The control chest X-ray after the procedure revealed the leads were in normal positions, as shown in Figure 7.

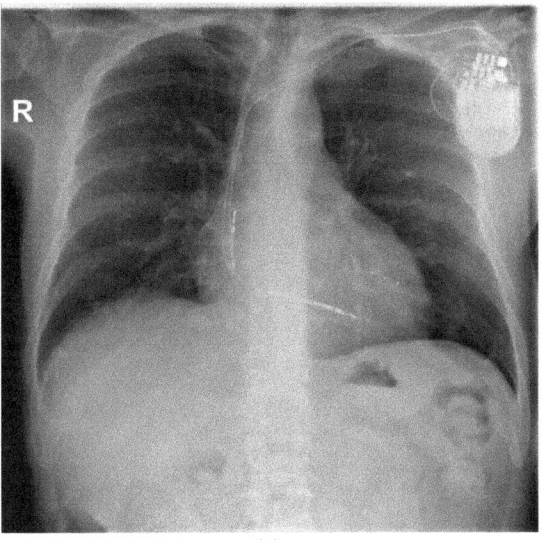
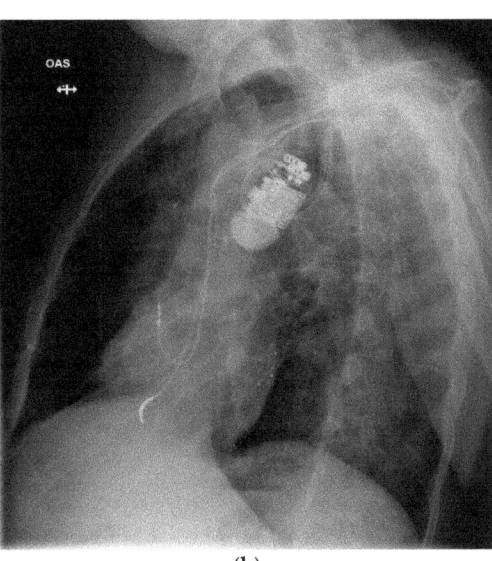

(a) (b)

Figure 7. CRT-D system with leads in normal positions: (**a**) posteroanterior view and (**b**) left anterior oblique view.

2.3. Third Clinical Case

2.3.1. Patient's Medical History and Presentation

A 37-year-old female patient, with a cardiac resynchronization therapy pacemaker (CRT-P), was admitted to the Cardiology Department for the extraction of magnetic resonance non-conditional leads and implantation of a new magnetic resonance (MR)-conditional CRT-P.

The patient is known to have had a surgical correction of atrial and ventricular septal defects at 18 years. Right after the surgery, she developed a complete AV block, and a pacemaker with single unipolar with a passive fixation lead (non-MR-conditional) was implanted on the right ventricle apex. At the age of 26, the pacemaker had been upgraded to a dual chamber pacemaker with the implantation of a bipolar active fixation lead (non-MR-conditional) in the right atrial appendage. Seven years after the upgrade to a dual chamber pacemaker, she was scheduled for a pacemaker replacement as the battery reached its elective replacement indicators (ERI). Since the patient complained about shortness of breath and fatigue at a moderate physical effort, and the ECG revealed a broad QRS complex with a left bundle branch block (LBBB)-like aspect, the decision to upgrade the system to CRT-P was made. A bipolar OTW (MR-conditional) was placed in the posterolateral vein. In 2020, she presented an epileptic seizure, a left frontal tumor was diagnosed on computed tomography, and MRI was recommended for a better evaluation and to establish the best neurosurgical approach.

At the time of admission to our department, the patient was asymptomatic. The ECG showed a sinus rhythm with biventricular paced activity triggered by the atrial activity. An echocardiogram revealed normal left ventricle function with preserved ejection fraction, mild tricuspid regurgitation, and no visible vegetations. A chest X-ray revealed a normal cardiothoracic ratio, a pulse generator PM placed subcutaneously in the left subclavian area, and three leads (as shown in Figure 8).

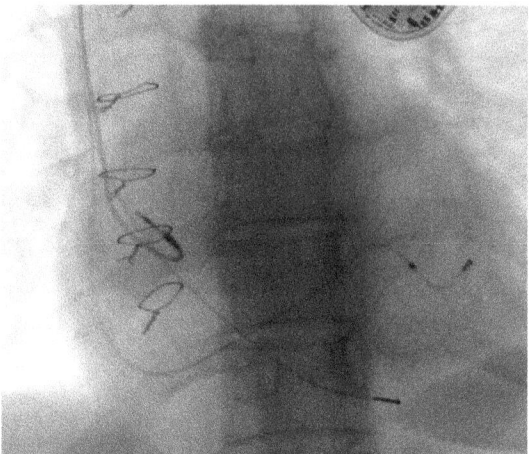

Figure 8. Chest X-ray at the time of admission at the hospital, with one lead positioned in the right atrial appendage, one on the apex of the right ventricle, and another one in the posterolateral vein.

Pacemaker interrogation revealed 100% ventricular paced and no underlying ventricular rhythm, with all leads having impedance, pacing, and sensing parameters within normal limits.

2.3.2. Transvenous Leads Extraction Procedure

Temporary cardiac pacing was performed by the right femoral vein approach, maintaining a stand-by heart rate of 50 beats/min, as the patient was pacemaker-dependent.

After deep analgesia-sedation, an incision was made, and the pulse generator was extracted. The three leads were disconnected and dissected up to the sutures to release them from the scar tissue. The unipolar, passive fixation RV lead was 20 years old; the RA bipolar, active fixation lead was 12 years old; and the LV bipolar, OTW lead was 5 years old. Gentle traction was made to mobilize the three leads, without the possibility of withdrawing them.

The connecter of the RA lead was cut off, and a Liberator locking stylet was advanced up to the top of the lead, locked at this level, and secured using a one-tie accessory. The RV and LV leads were secured with guidewires. With continuous traction, a 9 French bidirectional, rotational, mechanical lead-extraction sheath (Evolution RL, Cook Medical, USA) was advanced over the lead, up to the left innominate vein, where excessive fibrosis surrounded all three leads. The extraction sheath was advanced with difficulty, and the lead was extracted (as shown in Supplementary Video S5). The RV and LV leads were extracted using the same technique (Supplementary Video S6 and Supplementary Video S7, respectively). After removing the RV lead, the outer sheath was kept at the RA level. One 0.035″/180 cm J-tip guidewire was inserted in the RA through the outer sheath, being used to introduce the other two 0.038″/50 cm J-tip guidewires. Figure 9 shows the extracted leads with excessive fibrous tissue on the distal end of the RA and RV leads.

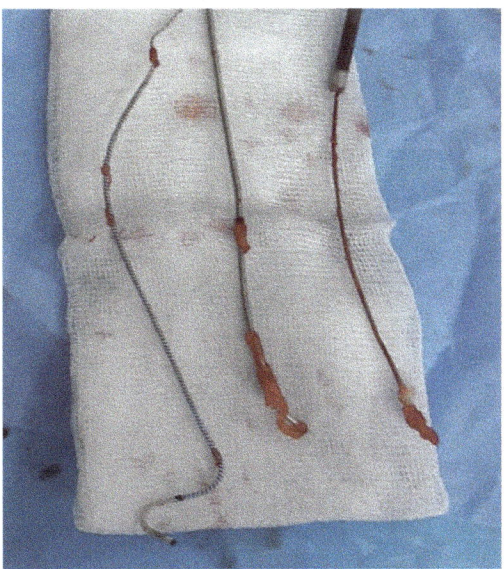

Figure 9. Extracted leads with excessive fibrous tissue on the distal end of RA and RV leads.

The 0.035″/180 cm J-tip guidewire was used to introduce a LV OTW BP lead through Biotronik Selectra Bio 2 45 cm sheath (Biotronik, Germany) in the posterolateral vein. The impedance, pacing, and sensing parameters were within normal limits, and the patient did not have phrenic stimulation at high voltage. The other guidewires were used to introduce an RV bipolar, active fixation lead on the apex of the RV and an RA bipolar active fixation lead on the right atrial appendage. All three leads were connected to a CRT pacemaker placed on the revised left pre-pectoral pocket. All three leads and the pacemaker are MRI compatible.

During the TLE procedure, the patient remained hemodynamically stable, and the echocardiography evaluation revealed no pericardial effusion, tricuspid valve lesions, or remaining lead fragments.

The overall fluoroscopy time for this procedure was 8 min.

One month later, the neurosurgical intervention was performed with complete macroscopic ablation of the left frontal tumor formation and gyral resection. Postoperative, periodic cerebral MRI investigations were required to monitor the patient's status.

3. Discussion

Transvenous lead extraction, the gold standard for lead removal, is a procedure that may involve several complications, so the decision to perform it must carefully weigh the risks and benefits. In this paper, we present three clinical cases of patients who presented different indications of TLE and explain how the procedures were successfully performed.

3.1. TLE Organizations and Security Measures

Due to organizational problems and economic issues, TLE centers use a different approach in the application of safety requirements; in some centers, the TLE procedure is performed in an electrophysiology, catheterization, or laboratory room, with deep analgesia-sedation, while in other centers, TLE is performed in an operating room/hybrid room, with general anesthesia and additional monitoring of the procedure (transesophageal echocardiography and arterial line), in the presence of a cardiac surgeon [10,11]. Transesophageal echocardiography, when used as a monitoring tool during TLE, was observed to provide higher rates of complete procedural success and a reduced risk of major complications [12].

The location where TLE procedure is performed is less important than the immediate availability of cardiothoracic surgical intervention. The time to surgical intervention is the most important factor in preventing death due to a major complication; therefore, organizational conditions should ensure the possibility of performing an emergency sternotomy within 5–10 min from the onset of the first symptoms of major complication [13,14].

Nowadays, personalized medicine, adapted to the particular situation of each patient, is the correct attitude. There are complex cases (with a large number of abandoned leads, very old leads, elderly or frail patients, and multiple comorbidities). In these situations, it is safer to start the procedure under general anesthesia and with transesophageal echocardiographic guidance. There are also cases, with only one or two leads to be extracted, in which general anesthesia and transesophageal ultrasound are usually not necessary during the procedure, knowing that many leads, especially those with a few years of dwell time, can be extracted by free traction without needing extraction materials. However, it is true that during the TLE procedure, the interventional team must have the ability to quickly change the work strategy depending on the case's evolution.

3.2. Particularities of the Cases

For the first clinical case, biochemical evaluation excluded systemic inflammation, and the blood cultures and wound-drainage cultures excluded local infection, but given the risk of underlying endocarditis, the pocket erosion associated with skin retraction was a clear indication for the total removal of the entire ICD system [15]. In this case, due to an abandoned lead in the tissues from many years ago, it was necessary to remove two dual-coil ICD leads. This complicated the procedure and extended the fluoroscopy time. Safe deactivation of the anti-tachycardia therapies of the ICD device was required before the procedure, since electrocautery was used close to the device. Electrocautery can cause electrical interference that may interfere with the function of implanted devices and, for patients with ICDs, it can even cause inappropriate internal electric shocks [16]. The extent and nature of the scar tissue structure in the CIED pocket walls was correlated with the relative position of cardiac lead loops concerning the device itself. Lead movements underneath the device can lead to pocket-wall irritation in the capsule-formation phase, resulting in more extensive scarring formation [17].

In the second case, the simple upgrade from a dual-chamber system to cardiac resynchronization therapy was initially desired, which would have involved only the introduction of a new lead for LV pacing. The impossibility of passing through the deep venous axis due to occlusion of the left subclavian vein during the procedure determined the decision to remove the RV lead and replace it with a single-coil defibrillation lead. In this way, all the guidelines' recommendations for patients with ischemic cardiomyopathy were fulfilled, knowing that CRT-D has been associated with a significant reduction in the risk of all-cause mortality compared with CRT-P in these patients [9].

Studies reported that total occlusion of the subclavian or brachiocephalic vein can occur on average in 12% (range 2–22%) of patients without an infection and with normally functioning leads [18]. Moreover, several hypotheses support the idea that more leads within a vein may be associated with a higher rate of occlusion [18]. Thus, this complication is not uncommon after CIED implantation [19]. In this case, the fluoroscopy time was slightly longer due to the complexity of the procedure. The outer sheath of the extraction system was kept at the RA level and used as a path for the two guidewires. They were utilized to introduce the single-coil defibrillation lead in the RV and to cannulate the coronary sinus for the LV lead.

The main interaction between the MRI and the non-MR-conditional pacemaker lead occurs due to the radiofrequency (RF) field generated by an MRI machine. If exposed to an MRI field, it causes adverse effects such as inappropriate device function due to interaction with the magnetic reed switch, device reset, pacing or sensing problems, changes in sensing or capture thresholds, and even lead perforation due to heating at the lead tip [9].

The advancement of MR-conditional technology has led to more complex clinical issues and better options for patient management. The current MR-conditional pacing technology provides solutions to some specific issues related to MR scanning [20]. In the case of the third patient, with repeated upgrades over time, the CRT pacemaker worked very well. However, the diagnosis of severe neurosurgical pathology required the replacement of the entire system with a new MRI-conditional one, to allow for a brain MRI examination and better management of the brain tumor. The TLE procedure was not without risks in a young patient who is completely pacemaker-dependent, but it was necessary and beneficial for MRI access, not only for the first evaluation before surgery but also for several periodic brain MRI investigations for follow-up.

It was reported that patients with a non-MRI-conditional CIED can perform an MRI at a field strength of 1.5 tesla without significant adverse events [21,22]. Even the current European Society of Cardiology guideline states that 1.5 tesla MRI scans (limited to SAR < 1.5 W/kg) may be considered in selected patients. The scans should be extrathoracic, and patients should not be pacemaker-dependent, taking into account the risk–benefit ratio of each patient [9]. For the patient in the third clinical case, a 3 tesla MRI brain examination was recommended for the evaluation of the tumor; since the patient was pacemaker-dependent, we decided to extract the leads and implant a new MR-conditional CRT-P, to avoid any risk during the MRI scanning or afterward.

Dual-coil leads are associated with more fibrosis and tissue in-growth, increasing the difficulty of extraction. The presence of two dual-coil implantable cardioverter-defibrillators causes significantly increased procedural risks [23].

Fibrotic scar tissue develops in areas where the leads are in contact with the endothelium. The first step is characterized by the thrombus formation along the lead at the time of implantation. The second step is characterized by the fibrosis of the thrombus resulting in almost complete encapsulation of the lead with a fibrin sheath, within 4–5 days of the implant procedure [24,25]. The venous entry site, the superior vena cava, and the electrode–endocardial interface are the most commons sites of adhesion formation [26]. In many patients, multiple areas of scar tissue are found, and this fibrotic tissue resists lead extraction, which may complicate the extraction procedure [27].

Increased precautions should be taken when scheduling patients with venous occlusion for TLE, as the lead extraction may be more difficult in these patients, requiring more advanced tools and more time. Older occlusions consisting of heavy fibrosis or even calcified tissue may require advanced extraction tools such as dilator sheaths and evolution sheaths [28].

Even if dual-coil leads are associated with greater procedural extraction risk due to fibrotic tissue in-growth into the proximal coil, another dual-coil lead was used in the first clinical case, since it provides superior defibrillation for a right-sided implant [29].

During extraction, uncoiling of the leads can happen, which results in retained components or failed extraction. To prevent this, a locking stylet was used to pull the lead from the tip and seal the tip of the lead during extraction. A one-tie compression coil was used for all procedures to aid in the removal of the lead, by binding the proximal components together and to the engaged locking stylet [23].

3.3. Advantages of Rotational, Mechanical Extraction Devices

The first generation of rotational, mechanical extraction devices had a unidirectional rotation mechanism, which was found to cause a phenomenon known as 'lead wrapping' in the presence of companion leads. Thus, the second generation of rotational, mechanical extraction devices have been designed to address this issue. The bidirectional, rotational mechanism seems to have a less aggressive tip, reducing the risk of damage to vascular structures, leads, or myocardial tissue [30].

Very commonly used bidirectional, rotational mechanism sheaths are the Evolution mechanical dilator sheath and TightRail™ mechanical dilator sheath.

The Evolution mechanical dilator sheath (Cook Medical, Bloomington, IN, USA) uses a rotational mechanism with a stainless-steel bladed tip to overcome fibrosis and cut adherences. The outer sheath covers the cutting edge when cutting activity is not desired, so venous walls are protected from damage. In addition, a shorter Evolution dilator sheath (Shortie) has been designed with a sharper blade to facilitate venous access in cases with extensive calcification under the clavicle [31].

The TightRail™ mechanical dilator sheath (Spectranetics Corp., Colorado Springs, CO, USA) has a more flexible shaft with a shielded metal blade at the distal tip. The flexible shaft facilitates progression through tortuous vascular structures and fibrotic and calcific attachments. Moreover, the dilating metal blade at the distal tip is shielded until activated [32].

Results from a multicenter Italian registry that enrolled 124 patients with 238 lead extracts reported a clinical success rate of 100%, with no deaths or major complications and only five minor complications (4%), when an Evolution R bidirectional, rotational mechanical lead-extraction sheath was used [30]. Other studies that evaluated the TightRail ™ reported the same kind of results. Choi et al. successfully and safely used a TightRail ™ Evolution R bidirectional, rotational, mechanical lead-extraction sheath to extract 131 leads from 86 patients, whose longest lead age was less than 10 years [33]. A more recent study by Mazzone et al. reported the safety and efficacy of the bidirectional, rotational, mechanical sheath TightRail™ for 57 lead extractions in 26 patients [34].

When comparing the two types of rotational, mechanical dilator sheaths regarding the efficacy and safety of transvenous lead extraction in different clinical indications for 163 lead extractions in 98 consecutive patients, the conclusion was that using the Evolution and the TightRail rotational, mechanical dilator sheaths was similarly effective and safe [35].

For all three cases presented, the fluoroscopy time was reduced. These bidirectional powered-extraction sheaths with rotating sharp blades at the tip are a safe method that allows for both fluoroscopy and the overall procedural time to be reduced and ensures better patient comfort [35].

3.4. Practical Approaches When Performing TLE Using Rotational, Mechanical Extraction Devices

In order to reduce the risk of complications during TLE procedures, we suggest paying special attention to the following steps:

- a contrast dye injection should be performed on the peripheral vein of the involved region to highlight the deep venous and collateral circulation;
- it is essential to insert the locking guide (locking-stylet type) up to the tip of the lead in order to stiffen the lead as much as possible;
- it is essential to always perform a light traction of the assembly that indicates use in the fixation areas: subclavian vein, left brachiocephalic vein or only at the tip of the lead in RA and RV;
- it is essential to choose the extraction sheath well, usually 2 French larger than the lead's diameter;
- it is essential to exert a continuous and constant traction force to achieve an optimal rotational sheath's rail, without rash tractions;
- in certain situations, it is profitable to use a short sheath and to release the lead at the level of the subclavian vein and the brachiocephalic vein, which should then be replaced with a long sheath in order to release the lead up to its tip;
- the use of a counterattraction sheath, handled by a second operator, might be useful to fix the fibrin ties and to facilitate their cutting as well as to prevent inversion of the ventricular wall at the lead's tip and to facilitate its release.

4. Conclusions

Transvenous lead extraction is regarded as the first-line strategy for the management of complications associated with cardiac implantable electronic devices when lead removal is indicated. The decision to perform a lead extraction should take into consideration not only the clinical indication for the procedure but also many other factors such as risks versus benefits, extractor and team experience, and even patient preference. Bidirectional, rotational mechanism sheaths can be safely used for these procedures.

Supplementary Materials: The following are available online at https://www.mdpi.com/article/10.3390/ijerph20010379/s1.

Author Contributions: Conceptualization, P.-M.B. and Ș.H.R.; methodology A.N.R.; software, I.D.P.; validation, Ș.H.R. and A.N.R.; formal analysis, C.A.T.; investigation, I.D.P.; resources, Ș.H.R.; data curation, P.-M.B.; writing—original draft preparation P.-M.B. and A.N.R.; writing—review and editing, Ș.H.R.; visualization, P.-M.B.; supervision, Ș.H.R.; project administration, C.A.T.; funding acquisition, Ș.H.R. All authors have read and agreed to the published version of the manuscript.

Funding: This research received no external funding.

Institutional Review Board Statement: The study was conducted according to the guidelines of the Declaration of Helsinki and was approved by the ethics committee of "Niculae Stăncioiu" Heart Institute, Cluj-Napoca (approval number 11568/09.11.2021).

Informed Consent Statement: Written informed consent was obtained from all patients for the publication of any potentially identifiable images or data included in this article.

Conflicts of Interest: The authors declare no conflict of interest.

References

1. Joy, P.S.; Kumar, G.; Poole, J.E.; London, B.; Olshansky, B. Cardiac implantable electronic device infections: Who is at greatest risk? *Heart Rhythm.* **2017**, *14*, 839–845. [CrossRef] [PubMed]
2. Azevedo, A.I.; Primo, J.; Gonçalves, H.; Oliveira, M.; Adão, L.; Santos, E.; Ribeiro, J.; Fonseca, M.; Dias, A.V.; Vouga, L.; et al. Lead extraction of cardiac rhythm Devices: A report of a single-center experience. *Front. Cardiovasc. Med.* **2017**, *4*, 18. [CrossRef] [PubMed]
3. Jacheć, W.; Polewczyk, A.; Polewczyk, M.; Tomasik, A.; Kutarski, A. Transvenous lead extraction SAFeTY score for risk stratification and proper patient selection for removal procedures using mechanical tools. *J. Clin. Med.* **2020**, *9*, 361. [CrossRef] [PubMed]
4. Perez, A.A.; Woo, F.W.; Tsang, D.C.; Carrillo, R.G. Transvenous lead extractions: Current approaches and future trends. *Arrhythm. Electrophysiol. Rev.* **2018**, *7*, 210–217. [CrossRef]
5. Tułecki, Ł.; Polewczyk, A.; Jacheć, W.; Nowosielecka, D.; Tomków, K.; Stefańczyk, P.; Kosior, J.; Duda, K.; Polewczyk, M.; Kutarski, A. A Study of Major and Minor Complications of 1500 Transvenous Lead Extraction Procedures Performed with Optimal Safety at Two High-Volume Referral Centers. *Int. J. Environ. Res. Public Health* **2021**, *18*, 10416. [CrossRef]
6. Tułecki, Ł.; Polewczyk, A.; Jacheć, W.; Nowosielecka, D.; Tomków, K.; Stefańczyk, P.; Kosior, J.; Duda, K.; Polewczyk, M.; Kutarski, A. Analysis of Risk Factors for Major Complications of 1500 Transvenous Lead Extraction Procedures with Especial Attention to Tricuspid Valve Damage. *Int. J. Environ. Res. Public Health* **2021**, *18*, 9100. [CrossRef]
7. Maytin, M.; Jones, S.O.; Epstein, L.M. Long-term mortality after transvenous lead extraction. *Circ. Arrhythm. Electrophysiol.* **2012**, *5*, 252–257. [CrossRef]
8. Nowosielecka, D.; Jacheć, W.; Polewczyk, A.; Tułecki, Ł.; Kleinrok, A.; Kutarski, A. Prognostic Value of Preoperative Echocardiographic Findings in Patients Undergoing Transvenous Lead Extraction. *Int. J. Environ. Res. Public Health* **2021**, *18*, 1862. [CrossRef]
9. Glikson, M.; Nielsen, J.C.; Kronborg, M.B.; Michowitz, Y.; Auricchio, A.; Barbash, I.M.; Barrabés, J.A.; Boriani, G.; Braunschweig, F.; Brignole, M.; et al. ESC Scientific Document Group. 2021 ESC Guidelines on cardiac pacing and cardiac resynchronization therapy: Developed by the Task Force on cardiac pacing and cardiac resynchronization therapy of the European Society of Cardiology (ESC) with the special contribution of the European Heart Rhythm Association (EHRA). *Eur. Heart J.* **2021**, *42*, 3427–3520. [CrossRef]
10. Stefańczyk, P.; Nowosielecka, D.; Tułecki, Ł.; Tomków, K.; Polewczyk, A.; Jacheć, W.; Kleinrok, A.; Borzęcki, W.; Kutarski, A. Transvenous Lead Extraction without Procedure-Related Deaths in 1000 Consecutive Patients: A Single-Center Experience. *Vasc. Health Risk Manag.* **2021**, *17*, 445–459. [CrossRef]

11. Kutarski, A.; Jacheć, W.; Polewczyk, A.; Nowosielecka, D.; Miszczak-Knecht, M.; Brzezinska, M.; Bieganowska, K. Transvenous Lead Extraction in Adult Patient with Leads Implanted in Childhood-Is That the Same Procedure as in Other Adult Patients? *Int. J. Environ. Res. Public Health* **2022**, *19*, 14594. [CrossRef] [PubMed]
12. Nowosielecka, D.; Jacheć, W.; Polewczyk, A.; Tułecki, Ł.; Tomków, K.; Stefańczyk, P.; Tomaszewski, A.; Brzozowski, W.; Szcześniak-Stańczyk, D.; Kleinrok, A.; et al. Transesophageal Echocardiography as a Monitoring Tool during Transvenous Lead Extraction—Does It Improve Procedure Effectiveness? *J. Clin. Med.* **2020**, *9*, 1382. [CrossRef]
13. Epstein, L.M.; Maytin, M. Strategies for transvenous lead extraction procedures. *J. Innov. Card. Rhythm Manag.* **2017**, *8*, 2702–2716. [CrossRef]
14. Boarescu, P.-M.; Roşian, A.-N.; Roşian, Ş.H. Transvenous Lead Extraction Procedure—Indications, Methods, and Complications. *Biomedicines* **2022**, *10*, 2780. [CrossRef] [PubMed]
15. Cassagneau, R.; Ploux, S.; Ritter, P.; Jan, E.; Barandon, L.; Deplagne, A.; Clementy, J.; Haïssaguerre, M.; Bordachar, P. Long-Term Outcomes after Pocket or Scar Revision and Reimplantation of Pacemakers with Preerosion. *Pacing Clin. Electrophysiol.* **2011**, *34*, 150–154. [CrossRef] [PubMed]
16. Doncaster and Bassetlaw Teaching Hospitals NHS Foundation Trust. Available online: https://www.dbth.nhs.uk/wp-content/uploads/2017/07/PAT-T-55-v-2-Deactivation-of-Implantable-Caradioverter-Defibrillator-and-CRT-Devices-Final.pdf (accessed on 28 October 2021).
17. Steckiewicz, R.; Świętoń, E.B.; Kołodzińska, A.; Bogdańska, M.; Solarz, P. Morphometric parameters of cardiac implantable electronic device (CIED) pocket walls observed on device replacement. *Folia Morphol.* **2017**, *76*, 675–681. [CrossRef]
18. Bracke, F.; Meijer, A.; Van Gelder, B. Venous occlusion of the access vein in patients referred for lead extraction: Influence of patient and lead characteristics. *Pacing Clin. Electrophysiol.* **2003**, *26*, 1649–1652. [CrossRef]
19. Czajkowski, M.; Jacheć, W.; Polewczyk, A.; Kosior, J.; Nowosielecka, D.; Tułecki, Ł.; Stefańczyk, P.; Kutarski, A. The Influence of Lead-Related Venous Obstruction on the Complexity and Outcomes of Transvenous Lead Extraction. *Int. J. Environ. Res. Public Health* **2021**, *18*, 9634. [CrossRef]
20. Shinbane, J.S.; Colletti, P.M.; Shellock, F.G. Magnetic resonance imaging in patients with cardiac pacemakers: Era of "MR Conditional" designs. *J. Cardiovasc. Magn. Reson.* **2011**, *13*, 63. [CrossRef]
21. Russo, R.J.; Costa, H.S.; Silva, P.D.; Anderson, J.L.; Arshad, A.; Biederman, R.W.; Boyle, N.G.; Frabizzio, J.V.; Birgersdotter-Green, U.; Higgins, S.L.; et al. Assessing the risks associated with MRI in patients with a pacemaker or defibrillator. *N. Engl. J. Med.* **2017**, *376*, 755–764. [CrossRef]
22. Nazarian, S.; Hansford, R.; Rahsepar, A.A.; Weltin, V.; McVeigh, D.; Gucuk Ipek, E.; Kwan, A.; Berger, R.D.; Calkins, H.; Lardo, A.C.; et al. Safety of magnetic resonance imaging in patients with cardiac devices. *N. Engl. J. Med.* **2017**, *377*, 2555–2564. [CrossRef] [PubMed]
23. Kalahasty, G.; Ellenbogen, K.A. ICD Lead Design and the Management of Patients with Lead Failure. *Card. Electrophysiol. Clin.* **2009**, *1*, 173–191. [CrossRef] [PubMed]
24. Keiler, J.; Schulze, M.; Sombetzki, M.; Heller, T.; Tischer, T.; Grabow, N.; Wree, A.; Bänsch, D. Neointimal fibrotic lead encapsulation–Clinical challenges and demands for implantable cardiac electronic devices. *J. Cardiol.* **2017**, *70*, 7–17. [CrossRef]
25. Kołodzińska, A.; Kutarski, A.; Koperski, Ł.; Grabowski, M.; Małecka, B.; Opolski, G. Differences in encapsulating lead tissue in patients who underwent transvenous lead removal. *Europace* **2012**, *14*, 994–1001. [CrossRef] [PubMed]
26. Smith, H.J.; Fearnot, N.E.; Byrd, C.L.; Wilkoff, B.L.; Love, C.J.; Sellers, T.D.; US Lead Extraction Database. Five-years experience with intravascular lead extraction. *Pacing Clin. Electrophysiol.* **1994**, *17*, 2016–2020. [CrossRef]
27. Koulouris, S.; Metaxa, S. Intravascular Lead Extractions: Tips and Tricks. In *Book Current Issues and Recent Advances in Pacemaker Therapy*; Roka, A., Ed.; IntechOpen: London, UK, 2012. Available online: https://www.intechopen.com/chapters/38318 (accessed on 28 October 2021).
28. Li, X.; Ze, F.; Wang, L.; Li, D.; Duan, J.; Guo, F.; Yuan, C.; Li, Y.; Guo, J. Prevalence of venous occlusion in patients referred for lead extraction: Implications for tool selection. *Europace* **2014**, *16*, 1795–1799. [CrossRef]
29. Swerdlow, C.D.; Kalahasty, G.; Ellenbogen, K.A. Implantable cardiac defibrillator lead failure and management. *J. Am. Coll. Cardiol.* **2016**, *67*, 1358–1368. [CrossRef]
30. Mazzone, P.; Migliore, F.; Bertaglia, E.; Facchin, D.; Daleffe, E.; Calzolari, V.; Crosato, M.; Melillo, F.; Peruzza, F.; Marzi, A.; et al. Safety and efficacy of the new bidirectional rotational Evolution® mechanical lead extraction sheath: Results from a multicentre Italian registry. *EP Europace* **2018**, *20*, 829–834. [CrossRef]
31. Hussein, A.A.; Wilkoff, B.L.; Martin, D.O.; Karim, S.; Kanj, M.; Callahan, T.; Baranowski, B.; Saliba, W.; Wazni, O. Initial experience with the Evolution mechanical dilator sheath for lead extraction: Safety and efficacy. *Heart Rhythm.* **2010**, *7*, 870–873. [CrossRef]
32. Aytemir, K.; Yorgun, H.; Canpolat, U.; Şahiner, M.L.; Kaya, E.B.; Evranos, B.; Özer, N. Initial experience with the TightRail™ Rotating Mechanical Dilator Sheath for transvenous lead extraction. *EP Europace* **2016**, *18*, 1043–1048. [CrossRef]
33. Choi, J.H.; Park, S.J.; Kim, H.R.; Kwon, H.J.; Park, K.M.; On, Y.K.; Kim, J.S.; Kim, J.Y.; Jung, W.Y. Transvenous lead extraction using the TightRail mechanical rotating dilator sheath for Asian patients. *Sci. Rep.* **2021**, *11*, 22251. [CrossRef] [PubMed]

34. Mazzone, P.; Melillo, F.; Radinovic, A.; Marzi, A.; Paglino, G.; Della Bella, P.; Mascioli, G. Use of the new rotating dilator sheath TightRail™ for lead extraction: A bicentric experience. *J. Arrhythm.* **2020**, *36*, 343–350. [CrossRef] [PubMed]
35. Cay, S.; Ozeke, O.; Ozcan, F.; Topaloglu, S.; Aras, D. Comparison of two types of rotational mechanical dilatator sheath: Evolution® and TightRail™. *Pacing Clin. Electrophysiol.* **2019**, *42*, 1226–1235. [CrossRef] [PubMed]

Disclaimer/Publisher's Note: The statements, opinions and data contained in all publications are solely those of the individual author(s) and contributor(s) and not of MDPI and/or the editor(s). MDPI and/or the editor(s) disclaim responsibility for any injury to people or property resulting from any ideas, methods, instructions or products referred to in the content.

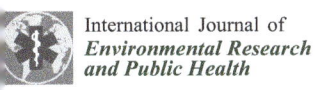

Article

Hemodynamic Effects of Permanent His Bundle Pacing Compared to Right Ventricular Pacing Assessed by Two-Dimensional Speckle-Tracking Echocardiography

Jedrzej Michalik [1], Alicja Dabrowska-Kugacka [2], Katarzyna Kosmalska [3], Roman Moroz [1], Adrian Kot [1], Ewa Lewicka [2] and Marek Szolkiewicz [1,*]

[1] Kashubian Center for Heart and Vascular Diseases, Department of Cardiology and Interventional Angiology, Pomeranian Hospitals, 84-200 Wejherowo, Poland; jedri1616@gmail.com (J.M.); romanmoroz@wp.pl (R.M.); aadriankot@gmail.com (A.K.)
[2] Department of Cardiology and Electrotherapy, Medical University of Gdansk, 80-214 Gdansk, Poland; alidab@gumed.edu.pl (A.D.-K.); ewa.lewicka@gumed.edu.pl (E.L.)
[3] Department of Cardiology, Pomeranian Hospitals, 81-348 Gdynia, Poland; katarzyn5@wp.pl
* Correspondence: e.mars@wp.pl

Citation: Michalik, J.; Dabrowska-Kugacka, A.; Kosmalska, K.; Moroz, R.; Kot, A.; Lewicka, E.; Szolkiewicz, M. Hemodynamic Effects of Permanent His Bundle Pacing Compared to Right Ventricular Pacing Assessed by Two-Dimensional Speckle-Tracking Echocardiography. *Int. J. Environ. Res. Public Health* **2021**, *18*, 11721. https://doi.org/10.3390/jerph182111721

Academic Editor: Paul B. Tchounwou

Received: 18 September 2021
Accepted: 6 November 2021
Published: 8 November 2021

Publisher's Note: MDPI stays neutral with regard to jurisdictional claims in published maps and institutional affiliations.

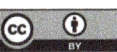

Copyright: © 2021 by the authors. Licensee MDPI, Basel, Switzerland. This article is an open access article distributed under the terms and conditions of the Creative Commons Attribution (CC BY) license (https://creativecommons.org/licenses/by/4.0/).

Abstract: We compared the effects of right ventricular (RVP; $n = 26$) and His bundle (HBP; $n = 24$) pacing in patients with atrioventricular conduction disorders and preserved LVEF. Postoperatively (1D), and after six months (6M), the patients underwent global longitudinal strain (GLS) and peak systolic dispersion (PSD) evaluation with 2D speckle-tracking echocardiography, assessment of left atrial volume index (LAVI) and QRS duration (QRSd), and sensing/pacing parameter testing. The RVP threshold was lower than the HBP threshold at 1D (0.65 ± 0.13 vs. 1.05 ± 0.20 V, $p < 0.001$), and then it remained stable, while the HBP threshold increased at 6M (1.05 ± 0.20 vs. 1.31 ± 0.30 V, $p < 0.001$). The RVP R-wave was higher than the HBP R-wave at 1D (11.52 ± 2.99 vs. 4.82 ± 1.41 mV, $p < 0.001$). The RVP R-wave also remained stable, while the HBP R-wave decreased at 6M (4.82 ± 1.41 vs. 4.50 ± 1.09 mV, $p < 0.02$). RVP QRSd was longer than HBP QRSd at 6M (145.0 ± 11.1 vs. 112.3 ± 9.3 ms, $p < 0.001$). The absolute value of RVP GLS decreased at 6M (16.32 ± 2.57 vs. $14.03 \pm 3.78\%$, $p < 0.001$), and HBP GLS remained stable. Simultaneously, RVP PSD increased (72.53 ± 24.15 vs. 88.33 ± 30.51 ms, $p < 0.001$) and HBP PSD decreased (96.28 ± 33.99 vs. 84.95 ± 28.98 ms, $p < 0.001$) after 6 months. RVP LAVI increased (26.73 ± 5.7 vs. 28.40 ± 6.4 mL/m^2, $p < 0.05$), while HBP LAVI decreased at 6M (30.03 ± 7.8 vs. 28.73 ± 8.7 mL/m^2, $p < 0.01$). These results confirm that HBP does not disrupt ventricular synchrony and provides advantages over RVP.

Keywords: His bundle pacing; ventricular synchrony; 2D speckle-tracking echocardiography; global longitudinal strain; left atrial volume

1. Introduction

Cardiac electrotherapy is a rapidly developing field of medicine. Modern biomedical technology provides opportunities to create devices that are small, durable and safe, with complex delivery systems or even leadless. Stimulation methods have also changed with the development of new technologies. Previously, we sought effective methods of stimulation, but we now seek methods that are both effective and physiological.

Right ventricular pacing (RVP) is common and easy to use. It requires no extraordinary surgical skills, allows practitioners to obtain adequate sensing and pacing parameters and causes minimal periprocedural complications. Unfortunately, it can cause both electrical and mechanical ventricular dyssynchrony, which diminishes the left ventricular (LV) function and may result in more frequent atrial fibrillation, heart failure and even death [1,2].

A significant milestone in electrotherapy was the introduction of biventricular stimulation, which partially restores the synchrony of contractions in both ventricles and improves

LV systolic function—benefits that are especially noticeable in patients with reduced LV ejection fraction (LVEF) and left bundle branch block. However, this method requires an additional pacing lead and is not suitable for all patients [3].

His bundle pacing (HBP), first described in 2000 by Deshmukh et al., appears to be the most physiological (and, therefore, optimal) form of cardiac stimulation. By pacing the native His-Purkinje system, HBP provides direct and synchronous stimulation of both ventricles [4,5]. Recent studies have shown that, although this is not a flawless method (it is technically difficult, generates low R-wave amplitudes, has a high rate of electrode dislocation and involves a high and often unstable stimulation threshold), it is feasible, produces a narrow QRS duration and prevents the development of pacing-induced cardiomyopathy [6]. Notably, in some cases, HBP efficiently corrects pre-existing bundle branch block, shortening the QRS duration and restoring the physiological synchrony of contractions [7].

Two-dimensional speckle-tracking echocardiography (2D STE) enables quantitative analysis of the degree of deformation in myocardial segments, as well as the scale of contraction dyssynchrony. Previous studies have shown that global longitudinal strain (GLS) and peak systolic dispersion (PSD) enable a more objective, accurate and reproducible assessment of myocardial dysfunction compared with tissue doppler imaging (TDI) or measurement of LVEF [8], which, so far, have been mainly used to assess the hemodynamic effects of HBP [9,10]. Left atrial volume is a recognised indicator of LV diastolic dysfunction, and it is a good predictor of atrial fibrillation [11]. The aim of this study was to analyse the safety and hemodynamic effects of chronic HBP compared with RVP using 2D STE.

2. Materials and Methods

This single-center, prospective, observational study was performed in Pomeranian hospitals. The participants ($n = 50$) were consecutive patients scheduled for permanent pacing therapy according to the current guidelines. The protocol was approved by the local ethics committee (KB-35/21) and all participants provided written informed consent. Patients at least 18 years of age, with a need for frequent ($\geq 70\%$) or continuous ventricular pacing, and with normal left ventricular systolic function (EF $\geq 50\%$) were considered for enrollment in the study. Exclusion criteria were chronic congestive heart failure, acute coronary syndrome, cardiomyopathy, advanced kidney or liver disease and any infectious disease. Patients with previously implanted cardiac pacing devices were also excluded.

Patients were divided into two groups: Group I ($n = 26$) underwent pacemaker implantation with RVP; Group II ($n = 24$) underwent pacemaker implantation with HBP. Right ventricular leads were implanted in standard mode. If required, the atrial lead was typically placed in the right atrial appendage. His bundle leads (Select Secure 3830, 69 cm, Medtronic Inc., Fridley, MN, USA) were placed with the appropriate delivery sheath (C315HIS, Medtronic Inc., Fridley, MN, USA) using an electrophysiology system for His potential mapping. Eight patients in Group I were diagnosed with permanent atrial fibrillation and high-degree atrio-ventricular block (AVB), and 18 were diagnosed with sinus rhythm and AVB. Thirteen patients in Group II were diagnosed with permanent atrial fibrillation and high-degree AVB, and 11 were diagnosed with sinus rhythm and AVB.

Pacing threshold and R-wave amplitude were recorded using the Medtronic system analyser (model 2090) immediately after the procedure (1D) and after six months (6M). QRS complex duration (QRSd) was obtained via electrophysiological equipment with electronic calipers at a sweep speed of 100 mm/s. QRSd was measured in lead V6 from the onset of intrinsic/paced QRS to the end of the QRS complex, before pacemaker implantation (0D), immediately after the procedure (1D) and at the 6-month follow-up visit (6M).

All patients underwent transthoracic echocardiography (VIVID S70 with M5Sc transducer, GE Healthcare System, Chicago, Il, USA) before, immediately after implantation (1D) and six months later (6M). This procedure was performed by one experienced sonographer (JM). Only echocardiograms of good quality and with frame rates between 40 and 80 frames per second were included for analysis. Left atrial volume index (LAVI) was calculated by dividing the endsystolic left atrial volume (measured with the area-length method) by the body surface area of patients. Estimation of global longitudinal peak systolic strain and peak systolic dispersion by 2D speckle tracking was performed in standard apical two-, three- and four-chamber views and calculated automatically (automated function imaging) offline using GE EchoPAC software (PC version 201). Moreover, AV delay was programmed postoperatively using echocardiography in order to provide the longest left ventricular diastolic filling time without atrial wave truncation, if applicable, separately for the sensed and the paced mode [12].

Statistical analysis was performed using IBM SPSS Statistics 18 software (SPSS Inc., Chicago, IL, USA) and Microsoft Excel 2007 software. Continuous data are expressed as mean ±SD, and the statistical significance of differences between the groups was assessed using the Student's t-test (or the Mann–Whitney test if the data were not normally distributed). Categorical data are expressed as percentages, and the statistical significance of differences between the groups was assessed using the χ^2 test. All p values under 0.05 were considered significant.

3. Results

The study cohort consisted of 50 consecutive patients (28 men and 22 women), randomly assigned to one of the two pacing sites. HBP was attempted in 26 patients; however, we failed in two cases, due to an unmappable His signal (1) and an unacceptably high His pacing threshold, respectively (1; overall success rate: 92%). In all, we included 24 patients with HBP (13 men and 11 women; 73.0 ± 14.4 years) and 26 with RVP (15 men and 11 women; 77.2 ± 6.7 years). All patients had high-degree atrioventricular conduction disorder, so we anticipated high rates of ventricular pacing (>70%). All the procedures were denovo implantations. Patient characteristics are presented in Table 1. There were no differences in demographic parameters, rates of comorbidities or indication for cardiac pacing between the groups.

Table 1. Clinical characteristics of patients with right ventricular pacing (RVP) and His bundle pacing (HBP).

	RVP (n = 26)	HBP (n = 24)	p-Value
Demographics			
Age (years)	77.2 ± 6.7	73.0 ± 14.4	n.s.
Sex (male, n/%)	15/58	13/54	n.s.
Indication for Pacing			
Sick Sinus Syndrome (n/%)	0/0	0/0	n.s.
Sinus Rhythm with AVB (n/%)	18/69	11/46	n.s.
Permanent Atrial Fibrillation with High-Degree AVB (n/%)	8/31	13/54	n.s.
Comorbidities			
Hypertension (n/%)	17/65	16/67	n.s.
Diabetes (n/%)	11/42	8/33	n.s.
Coronary Artery Disease (n/%)	8/31	6/25	n.s.
Chronic Kidney Disease (n/%)	8/31	5/21	n.s.
Atrial Fibrillation (n/%)	10/38	17/71	n.s.
LBBB/RBBB (n/%)	1/4	6/25	n.s.

At baseline (0D), RVP QRSd was shorter than HBP QRSd (108.1 ± 15.6 vs. 121.7 ± 23.4 ms, $p < 0.05$), but it significantly increased immediately after pacemaker implantation (108.1 ± 15.6 vs. 143.4 ± 9.2 ms, $p < 0.001$) and over the following six months (108.1 ± 15.6 vs. 145.0 ± 11.1 ms, $p < 0.001$). HBP QRSd did not significantly change during this time (121.7 ± 23.4 vs. 112.3 ± 9.3 ms, n.s.). In the 6-month follow-up visit, RVP QRSd was noticeably longer than HBP QRSd (145.0 ± 11.1 vs. 112.3 ± 9.3 ms, $p < 0.001$). These data are presented in Figure 1. The 12-lead ECG data of selected pacing are presented in Figure 2.

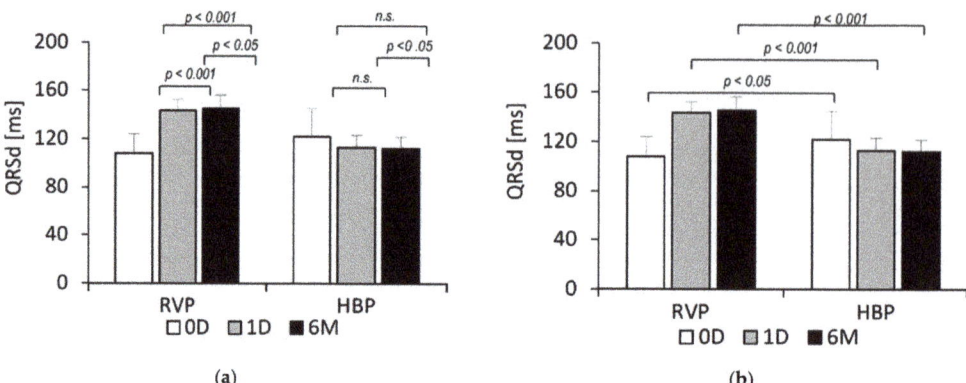

Figure 1. QRS complex duration (QRSd) in patients with right ventricular pacing (RVP) and His bundle pacing (HBP), at baseline (0D), immediately after pacemaker implantation (1D) and 6 months later (6M). Statistical analysis presented: (**a**) within and (**b**) between the studied groups of patients.

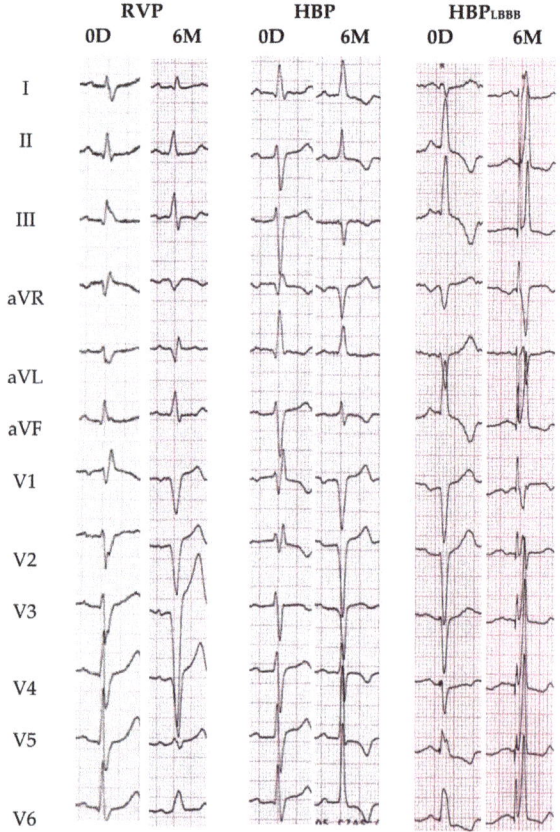

Figure 2. Comparison of 12-lead ECG recorded at a sweep speed of 25 mm/s before (0D) and 6 months after (6M) pacemaker implantation in selected patients treated with right ventricular pacing (RVP), His bundle pacing (HBP) and His bundle pacing in patients with pre-existing LBBB (HBP$_{LBBB}$).

There were significant differences in pacing threshold and R-wave amplitude between the RVP and HBP groups (Table 2). Immediately after pacemaker implantation (1D), the pacing threshold in the RVP group was lower than in the HBP group (0.65 ± 0.13 vs. 1.05 ± 0.20 V, $p < 0.001$); then, it remained stable until the 6-month follow-up visit. Meanwhile, the pacing threshold in the HBP group significantly increased (1.05 ± 0.20 vs. 1.31 ± 0.30 V, $p < 0.001$). The R-wave amplitude measured at 1D was higher in the RVP group than in the HBV group (11.52 ± 2.99 vs. 4.82 ± 1.41 mV, $p < 0.001$). It also remained stable until the 6-month follow-up visit, while the R-wave amplitude in the HBP group significantly decreased (4.82 ± 1.41 vs. 4.50 ± 1.09 mV, $p < 0.02$).

Table 2. Comparison of selected variables between (and within) RVP and HBP groups of patients immediately after pacemaker implantation (1D) and at 6-month follow-up visit (6M). Abbreviations: RVP—right ventricular pacing; HBV—His bundle pacing; GLS—global longitudinal strain; PSD—peak systolic dispersion; LAVI—left atrial volume index.

	RVP_{1D}	HBP_{1D}	p-Value	RVP_{1D}	RVP_{6M}	p-Value	HBP_{1D}	HBP_{6M}	p-Value	RVP_{6M}	HBP_{6M}	p-Value
Threshold (V)	0.65 ± 0.1	1.05 ± 0.2	<0.001	0.65 ± 0.1	0.66 ± 0.2	n.s.	1.05 ± 0.2	1.31 ± 0.3	<0.001	0.66 ± 0.2	1.31 ± 0.3	<0.001
R-wave (mV)	11.52 ± 3.0	4.82 ± 1.4	<0.001	11.52 ± 3.0	11.41 ± 2.3	n.s.	4.82 ± 1.4	4.50 ± 1.1	<0.02	11.41 ± 2.3	4.50 ± 1.1	<0.001
GLS (-%)	16.32 ± 2.6	14.85 ± 2.5	=0.051	16.32 ± 2.6	14.03 ± 3.8	<0.001	14.85 ± 2.5	14.98 ± 2.0	n.s.	14.03 ± 3.8	14.98 ± 2.0	n.s.
PSD (ms)	72.53 ± 24.2	96.28 ± 34.0	<0.01	72.53 ± 24.2	88.33 ± 30.5	<0.001	96.28 ± 34.0	84.95 ± 29.0	<0.001	88.33 ± 30.5	84.95 ± 29.0	n.s.
LAVI (mL/m^2)	26.73 ± 5.7	30.03 ± 7.8	n.s.	26.73 ± 5.7	28.40 ± 6.4	<0.05	30.03 ± 7.8	28.73 ± 8.7	<0.01	28.40 ± 6.4	28.73 ± 8.7	n.s.

Postoperatively (1D), the absolute value of global longitudinal strain (GLS) was greater in the RVP group than in the HBP group (Table 2); however, this difference fell slightly short of significance (16.32 ± 2.57 vs. 14.85 ± 2.52%, $p = 0.051$). After six months, GLS significantly decreased in the RVP group (16.32 ± 2.57 vs. 14.03 ± 3.78%, $p < 0.001$) and remained stable in the HBP group. No significant difference was found in GLS between the two groups six months after pacemaker implantation (14.03 ± 3.78 vs. 14.98 ± 1.96%, n.s.). Additionally, we analysed whether there were any differences in GLS between patients with sinus rhythm and AVB (SR+AVB) vs. patients with atrial fibrillation and AVB (AF+AVB). Postoperatively (1D), the absolute value of GLS in the RVP group was greater in the SR+AVB patients than in the patients with AF+AVB (16.93 ± 2.5 vs. 14.7 ± 2.1%, $p < 0.05$), and this difference was maintained after 6 months of follow-up (15.00 ± 3.5 vs. 11.68 ± 3.3%, $p < 0.05$). There were no significant differences in the absolute value of GLS SR+AVB vs. AF+AVB in the HBP group at 1D or 6M. It is worth noting that the absolute value of GLS in the RVP group decreased over 6 months in both SR+AVB and AF+AVB patients (16.93 ± 2.5 vs. 15.00 ± 3.5%, $p < 0.005$; 14.70 ± 2.1 vs. 11.68 ± 3.3%, $p < 0.005$; respectively), while it remained stable in both analysed groups of patients if the His bundle was paced. The data are presented in Table 3.

Table 3. Comparison of global longitudinal strain (GLS) between patients with sinus rhythm and atrioventricular block (SR+AVB) vs. patients with atrial fibrillation and atrioventricular block (AF+AVB) immediately after pacemaker implantation (1D) and at 6-month follow-up visit (6M). Abbreviations: RVP—right ventricular pacing; HBV—His bundle pacing.

	1D	6M	p-Value
RVP (SR+AVB)	16.93 ± 2.5	15.00 ± 3.5	<0.005
RVP (AF+AVB)	14.70 ± 2.1	11.68 ± 3.3	<0.005
p-value	<0.05	<0.05	
HBP (SR+AVB)	14.37 ± 2.9	15.20 ± 2.1	n.s.
HBP (AF+AVB)	15.76 ± 2.3	15.18 ± 1.9	n.s.
p-value	n.s.	n.s.	

Immediately after implantation (1D), peak systolic dispersion (PSD) was greater in the HBP group than in the RVP group (96.28 ± 33.99 vs. 72.53 ± 24.15 ms, $p < 0.01$). After six months, PSD significantly increased in the RVP group (72.53 ± 24.15 vs. 88.33 ± 30.51 ms, $p < 0.001$) and significantly decreased in the HBP group (96.28 ± 33.99 vs. 84.95 ± 28.98 ms,

$p < 0.001$). No significant difference was found in PSD between the two groups at the six-month follow-up visit (88.33 ± 30.51 vs. 84.95 ± 28.98 ms, n.s.). The data are presented in Table 2. GLS and PSD bull's eye diagrams are presented in Figure 3.

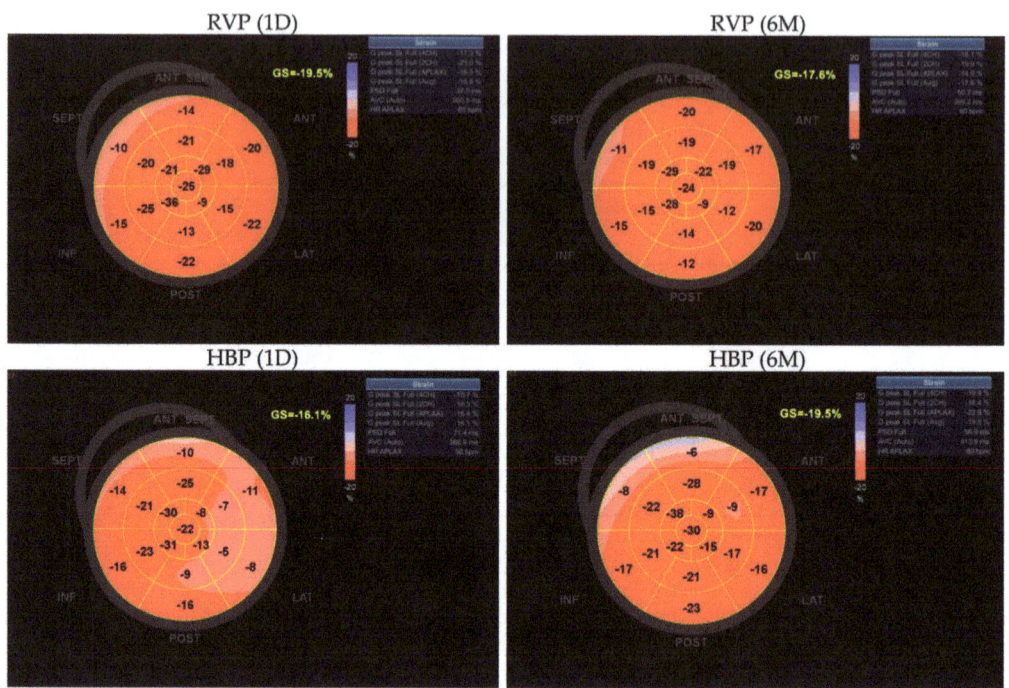

Figure 3. Echocardiographic assessment of left ventricular function using 2D speckle-tracking technique: bull's eye diagram of global longitudinal strain and peak systolic dispersion of selected patients with right ventricular pacing (RVP) and His bundle pacing (HBP) obtained immediately after pacemaker implantation (1D) and at 6-month follow-up visit (6M).

The left atrial volume index (LAVI) was also measured (Table 2). There was no difference in LAVI between the two groups postoperatively (26.73 ± 5.7 vs. 30.03 ± 7.8 mL/m^2, n.s.). Over the next six months, LAVI in the RVP group significantly increased (26.73 ± 5.7 vs. 28.40 ± 6.4 mL/m^2, $p < 0.05$), while it significantly decreased in the HBP group (30.03 ± 7.8 vs. 28.73 ± 8.7 mL/m^2, $p < 0.01$). However, there was still no difference between the groups at the 6-month follow-up visit (28.40 ± 6.4 vs. 28.73 ± 8.7 mL/m^2, n.s.).

4. Discussion

HBP is a natural step in the development of cardiac electrotherapy that enables the physiological stimulation of the heart. Recent research has demonstrated that HBP is justified both theoretically and practically. Physiological stimulation of the heart is supposed to improve electrocardiographic and echocardiographic parameters and provide beneficial effects in terms of quality of life, morbidity and even mortality. We demonstrated that HBP provides significant benefits over the commonly used RVP in terms of its electrocardiographic and echocardiographic parameters, which can be assumed to improve quality of life and reduce morbidity and mortality over the long term.

HBP is assumed to be more difficult to install than RVP, and, furthermore, HBP's achieved pacing/sensing parameters are worse than RVP's. Our results confirm these assumptions. The stimulation threshold in the HBP group immediately after implantation was fully acceptable, but it was higher than the RVP group's pacing threshold. Moreover, this threshold increased slightly over the six-month follow-up period, while it remained stable in the RVP group. The R-wave in the RVP group was also high and stable. In the HBP group, the R-wave was significantly lower immediately after the procedure, and it decreased further after six months. Similar differences were noticed in previous studies [13,14]. Group differences in the observed values do not, however, arouse any practical concern. While the above data are more favourable in the RVP group, which could be better in terms of pacemaker battery life, the data from both groups fall within ranges that ensure safe and effective pacing. However, the expected clinical benefits should outweigh the risk of greater energy loss and presumably faster battery consumption.

Electromechanical left ventricular systolic dyssynchrony causes most of the negative consequences associated with RVP, including pacing-induced cardiomyopathy [15]. This is not a common phenomenon in cardiac electrotherapy, but it is one of the most important reasons that researchers have focused more on physiological stimulation. QRSd is a good indicator of electrical synchrony. Our results show that, unlike RVP, HBP does not disrupt QRSd, triggering a simultaneous depolarization of the ventricles. QRSd in the RVP group significantly increased immediately after the procedure and (although less significantly) over the following six months. On the other hand, QRSd in the HBP group did not change significantly after the procedure, remaining relatively stable throughout the observation period. The stimulation mode influenced not only electrical but also mechanical synchrony, as evidenced by the peak systolic dispersion (PSD) measurements obtained using 2D STE. PSD adequately reflects the degree of mechanical dyssynchrony accompanying electrotherapy [16] and is used to assess left ventricular dysfunction in other pathologies as well [17,18]. Our PSD results are consistent with our findings for QRSd. During the six months of follow-up, PSD in the RVP group significantly increased, along with the prolonged QRSd, indicating electromechanical dyssynchrony in these patients. On the other hand, PSD in the HBP group significantly decreased. Similar conclusions have been presented in previous studies. Tang et al. showed a significantly greater PSD in the RVP group than in the HBP group as early as one week after the procedure [14]. Sun et al. observed significantly greater PSD values in the RVP group compared with the left bundle branch pacing (LBBP) group [19]. Bednarek et al. noted higher PSD values in patients with nonselective LBBP compared with patients with selective LBBP [16]. These studies support the hypothesis that the more physiological the stimulation, the lower the PSD values (thus, the lower the mechanical dyssynchrony).

Global longitudinal strain (GLS) is currently perceived as a highly valuable tool for assessing myocardial contractility disorders, much more sensitive than LVEF [8,20]. It is a good predictor of adverse events in patients with heart failure [21]. Studies show that the absolute value of GLS is significantly reduced when RVP is used [22]; GLS helps to predict the development of pacing-induced ventricular dysfunction [23]. Prakash et al. showed that GLS did not change during the six-month follow-up in patients with HBP, regardless of whether HBP was selective or nonselective [24]. In a study by Fehske et al., GLS in the RVP group was significantly reduced, while GLS in the HBV group did not change [25]. Our study corroborates these findings. GLS decreased significantly in the RVP group and did not change in the HBP group. There was no significant difference between the groups at the 6-month follow-up visit. We assume that extending the observation period would allow us to obtain a statistically significant difference. The observed effects were similar in patients with both sinus rhythm and permanent atrial fibrillation.

RVP adversely affects the structure and function of the left atrium [26]. In this study, we compared changes in LAVI, which reflect LV diastolic dysfunction. Increased LAVI is also a risk factor for the development of atrial fibrillation [11,27]. LAVI increased significantly in the RVP group and decreased in the HBP group. Pastore et al. also noted that RVP resulted in increased left atrial volume parameters compared with HBP [28]. This is another important feature of the hemodynamic disruptions accompanying RVP—one that can be avoided by changing the method of stimulation. Further studies are necessary to determine whether this intervention leads to a reduction in the incidence of clinical atrial fibrillation.

5. Limitations of the Study

This was a prospective, observational study with all the limitations characteristic for single-center studies. The number of patients and follow-up duration were limited and therefore the results should be interpreted with caution. Nevertheless, we demonstrated that HBP, when compared to RVP, maintains electrical and mechanical ventricular synchrony, preventing heart muscle systolic and diastolic function disorders. A larger, randomized, multicenter trial comparing RVP to HBP, with long-term follow-up, is necessary to confirm our findings.

6. Conclusions

The present study confirms the feasibility of HBP, with a high success rate (92%). This method provides adequate pacing and sensing parameters. Above all, unlike RVP, HBP does not disrupt electrical and mechanical ventricular synchrony, which can prevent the remodeling of the heart muscle that leads to systolic and diastolic dysfunction disorders. Thus, HBP maintains the hemodynamic balance, the lack of which leads to arrhythmias, heart failure and an increase in mortality. It is expected that, in the coming years, HBP/LBBP will become a commonly used method of cardiac pacing.

Author Contributions: Conceptualisation: A.D.-K., E.L. and M.S.; Formal analysis: J.M., A.D.-K., K.K., R.M., A.K., E.L. and M.S.; Investigation: J.M., K.K., A.K. and A.D.-K.; Methodology: J.M., K.K., R.M. and A.K.; Project administration: M.S.; Visualisation: J.M.; Writing—original draft: J.M.; Writing—review and editing: M.S.; Supervision: E.L. and M.S. All authors have read and agreed to the published version of the manuscript.

Funding: This research received no external funding.

Institutional Review Board Statement: The study was conducted according to the guidelines of the Declaration of Helsinki and approved by the Ethics Committee at the Regional Medical Chamber in Gdansk (KB-35/21).

Informed Consent Statement: Informed consent was obtained from all subjects involved in the study.

Data Availability Statement: The data supporting the findings of the study are available from Jedrzej Michalik (jedri33@gmail.com) on reasonable request.

Conflicts of Interest: The authors declare no conflict of interest.

References

1. Yu, C.-M.; Chan, J.Y.-S.; Zhang, Q.; Omar, R.; Yip, G.W.-K.; Hussin, A.; Fang, F.; Lam, K.H.; Chan, H.C.-K.; Fung, J.W.-H. Biventricular Pacing in Patients with Bradycardia and Normal Ejection Fraction. *N. Engl. J. Med.* **2009**, *361*, 2123–2134. [CrossRef]
2. Sweeney, M.O.; Hellkamp, A.S.; Ellenbogen, K.A.; Greenspon, A.J.; Freedman, R.A.; Lee, K.L.; Lamas, G.A. Adverse Effect of Ventricular Pacing on Heart Failure and Atrial Fibrillation Among Patients With Normal Baseline QRS Duration in a Clinical Trial of Pacemaker Therapy for Sinus Node Dysfunction. *Circulation* **2003**, *107*, 2932–2937. [CrossRef]
3. Ponikowski, P.; Voors, A.A.; Anker, S.D.; Bueno, H.; Cleland, J.G.F.; Coats, A.J.S.; Falk, V.; Gonzalez-Juanatey, J.R.; Harjola, V.P.; Jankowska, E.A.; et al. 2016 ESC Guidelines for the diagnosis and treatment of acute and chronic heart failure: The Task Force for the diagnosis and treatment of acute and chronic heart failure of the European Society of Cardiology (ESC) Developed with the special contribution of the Heart Failure Association (HFA) of the ESC. *Eur. Heart J.* **2016**, *37*, 2129–2200.
4. Vijayaraman, P.; Dandamudi, G.; Zanon, F.; Sharma, P.S.; Tung, R.; Huang, W.; Koneru, J.; Tada, H.; Ellenbogen, K.A.; Lustgarten, D.L. Permanent His bundle pacing: Recommendations from a Multicenter His Bundle Pacing Collaborative Working Group for standardization of definitions, implant measurements, and follow-up. *Heart Rhythm.* **2018**, *15*, 460–468. [CrossRef]
5. Deshmukh, P.; Casavant, D.A.; Romanyshyn, M.; Anderson, K. Permanent, direct His-bundle pacing: A novel approach to cardiac pacing in patients with normal His-Purkinje activation. *Circulation* **2000**, *101*, 869–877. [CrossRef]
6. Vijayaraman, P.; Chung, M.K.; Dandamudi, G.; Upadhyay, G.A.; Krishnan, K.; Crossley, G.; Campbell, K.B.; Lee, B.K.; Refaat, M.M.; Saksena, S.; et al. ACC's Electrophysiology Council: His Bundle Pacing. *J. Am. Coll. Cardiol.* **2018**, *72*, 927–947. [CrossRef] [PubMed]
7. Arnold, A.; Shun-Shin, M.J.; Keene, D.; Howard, J.P.; Sohaib, S.A.; Wright, I.J.; Cole, G.D.; Qureshi, N.A.; Lefroy, D.C.; Koa-Wing, M.; et al. His Resynchronization versus Biventricular Pacing in Patients with Heart Failure and Left Bundle Branch Block. *J. Am. Coll. Cardiol.* **2018**, *72*, 3112–3122. [CrossRef] [PubMed]

8. Luis, S.A.; Chan, J.; Pellikka, P.A. Echocardiographic Assessment of Left Ventricular Systolic Function: An Overview of Contemporary Techniques, Including Speckle-Tracking Echocardiography. *Mayo Clin. Proc.* **2019**, *94*, 125–138. [CrossRef] [PubMed]
9. Kronborg, M.B.; Mortensen, P.T.; Poulsen, S.H.; Gerdes, J.C.; Jensen, H.K.; Nielsen, J.C. His or para-His pacing preserves left ventricular function in atrioventricular block: A double-blind, randomized, crossover study. *Europace* **2014**, *16*, 1189–1196. [CrossRef]
10. Liu, X.; Li, W.; Wang, L.; Tian, S.; Zhou, X.; Wu, M. Safety and efficacy of left bundle branch pacing in comparison with conventional right ventricular pacing: A systematic review and meta-analysis. *Medicine* **2021**, *100*, e26560. [CrossRef]
11. Fatema, K.; Barnes, M.E.; Bailey, K.R.; Abhayaratna, W.P.; Cha, S.; Seward, J.B.; Tsang, T.S. Minimum vs. maximum left atrial volume for prediction of first atrial fibrillation or flutter in an elderly cohort: A prospective study. *Eur. J. Echocardiogr.* **2009**, *10*, 282–286. [CrossRef]
12. Antonini, L.; Auriti, A.; Pasceri, V.; Meo, A.; Pristipino, C.; Varveri, A.; Greco, S.; Santini, M. Optimization of the atrioventricular delay in sequential and biventricular pacing: Physiological bases, critical review, and new purposes. *Europace* **2012**, *14*, 929–938. [CrossRef]
13. Jastrzębski, M.; Moskal, P.; Bednarek, A.; Kiełbasa, G.; Czarnecka, D. His-bundle pacing as a standard approach in patients with permanent atrial fibrillation and bradycardia. *Pacing Clin. Electrophysiol.* **2018**, *41*, 1508–1512. [CrossRef]
14. Tang, J.; Chen, S.; Liu, L.; Liao, H.; Zhan, X.; Wu, S.; Liang, Y.; Chen, O.; Lin, C.; Zhang, Q.; et al. Assessment of Permanent Selective His Bundle Pacing in Left Ventricular Synchronization Using 3-D Speckle Tracking Echocardiography. *Ultrasound Med. Biol.* **2019**, *45*, 385–394. [CrossRef]
15. Kaye, G.; Ng, J.Y.; Ahmed, S.; Valencia, D.; Harrop, D.; Ng, A.C. The Prevalence of Pacing-Induced Cardiomyopathy (PICM) in Patients with Long Term Right Ventricular Pacing—Is it a Matter of Definition? *Heart Lung Circ.* **2019**, *28*, 1027–1033. [CrossRef] [PubMed]
16. Bednarek, A.; Ionita, O.; Moskal, P.; Linkova, H.; Kiełbasa, G.; Prochazkova, R.; Vesela, J.; Rajzer, M.; Curila, K.; Jastrzębski, M. Nonselective versus selective His bundle pacing: An acute intrapatient speckle-tracking strain echocardiographic study. *J. Cardiovasc. Electrophysiol.* **2021**, *32*, 117–125. [CrossRef]
17. Jalanko, M.; Tarkiainen, M.; Sipola, P.; Jääskeläinen, P.; Lauerma, K.; Laine, M.; Nieminen, M.S.; Laakso, M.; Heliö, T.; Kuusisto, J. Left ventricular mechanical dispersion is associated with nonsustained ventricular tachycardia in hypertrophic cardiomyopathy. *Ann. Med.* **2016**, *48*, 417–427. [CrossRef]
18. Li, C.; Yuan, M.; Li, K.; Bai, W.; Rao, L. Value of peak strain dispersion in discovering left ventricular dysfunction in diabetes mellitus. *Sci. Rep.* **2020**, *10*, 21437. [CrossRef]
19. Sun, Z.; Di, B.; Gao, H.; Lan, D.; Peng, H. Assessment of ventricular mechanical synchronization after left bundle branch pacing using 2-D speckle tracking echocardiography. *Clin. Cardiol.* **2020**, *43*, 1562–1572. [CrossRef]
20. Marwick, T.H.; Shah, S.J.; Thomas, J.D. Myocardial strain in the assessment of patients with heart failure: A review. *JAMA Cardiol.* **2019**, *4*, 287–294. [CrossRef]
21. Sengeløv, M.; Jørgensen, P.G.; Jensen, J.S.; Bruun, N.E.; Olsen, F.J.; Fritz-Hansen, T.; Nochioka, K.; Biering-Sørensen, T. Global Longitudinal Strain Is a Superior Predictor of All-Cause Mortality in Heart Failure With Reduced Ejection Fraction. *JACC Cardiovasc. Imaging* **2015**, *8*, 1351–1359. [CrossRef] [PubMed]
22. Saito, M.; Kaye, G.; Negishi, K.; Linker, N.; Gammage, M.; Kosmala, W.; Marwick, T.H. Dyssynchrony, contraction efficiency and regional function with apical and non-apical RV pacing. *Heart* **2015**, *101*, 600–608. [CrossRef]
23. Xu, H.; Li, J.; Bao, Z.; Xu, C.; Zhang, Y.; Liu, H.; Yang, J. Early Change in Global Longitudinal Strain is an Independent Predictor of Left Ventricular Adverse Remodelling in Patients with Right Ventricular Apical Pacing. *Heart Lung Circ.* **2019**, *28*, 1780–1787. [CrossRef] [PubMed]
24. Prakash, V.; Hegde, A.V.; Nagamalesh, U.; Ramkumar, S.; Krishnab, Y.S.; Prakashb, V.R.; Potlurib, A.R. His bundle pacing—Is it the final frontier of physiological pacing?–A single centre experience from the Indian sub–Continent. *Indian Heart J.* **2020**, *72*, 160–165. [CrossRef] [PubMed]
25. Fehske, W.; Israel, C.W.; Winter, S.; Ghorbany, P.; Nguyen, D.Q.; Voigt, J.U. Echocardiographic assessment of myocardial function during His bundle and right ventricular pacing. *Herzschrittmacherther. Elektrophysiol.* **2020**, *31*, 151–159. [CrossRef] [PubMed]
26. Xie, J.; Fang, F.; Zhang, Q.; Sanderson, J.; Chan, J.Y.-S.; Lam, Y.; Yu, C. Acute Effects of Right Ventricular Apical Pacing on Left Atrial Remodeling and Function. *Pacing Clin. Electrophysiol.* **2012**, *35*, 856–862. [CrossRef] [PubMed]
27. Tsang, T.S.; Gersh, B.J.; Appleton, C.P.; Tajik, A.J.; Barnes, M.E.; Bailey, K.R.; Oh, J.K.; Leibson, C.; Montgomery, S.C.; Seward, J.B. Left ventricular diastolic dysfunction as a predictor of the first diagnosed non-valvular atrial fibrillation in 840 elderly men and women. *J. Am. Coll. Cardiol.* **2002**, *40*, 1636–1644. [CrossRef]
28. Pastore, G.; Aggio, S.; Baracca, E.; Fraccaro, C.; Picariello, C.; Roncon, L.; Corbucci, G.; Noventa, F.; Zanon, F. Hisian area and right ventricular apical pacing differently affect left atrial function: An intra-patients evaluation. *Europace* **2014**, *16*, 1033–1039. [CrossRef]

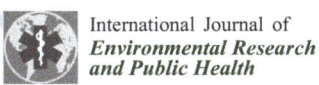

Case Report

Right Ventricular Endocardial Mapping and a Potential Arrhythmogenic Substrate in Cardiac Amyloidosis—Role of ICD

Aleksandra Liżewska-Springer [1,*], Tomasz Królak [1], Karolina Dorniak [2], Maciej Kempa [1], Alicja Dąbrowska-Kugacka [1], Grzegorz Sławiński [1] and Ewa Lewicka [1]

1. Department of Cardiology and Electrotherapy, Medical University of Gdansk, 80-952 Gdansk, Poland; tomasz.krolak@gumed.edu.pl (T.K.); maciej.kempa@gumed.edu.pl (M.K.); alidab@gumed.edu.pl (A.D.-K.); lek.grzegorzslawinski@gmail.com (G.S.); elew@gumed.edu.pl (E.L.)
2. Department of Nonivasive Cardiac Diagnostics, Medical University of Gdansk, 80-952 Gdansk, Poland; karolina.dorniak@gumed.edu.pl
* Correspondence: ollizz@gumed.edu.pl

Abstract: Patients with cardiac amyloidosis (CA) have an increased risk of sudden cardiac death (SCD). However, the role of an implantable cardioverter-defibrillator in the primary prevention of SCD in this group of patients is still controversial. We present a case with CA with recurrent syncope and non-sustained ventricular tachycardia. In order to further stratify the risk of SCD, an electrophysiological study with endocardial electroanatomic voltage mapping was performed prior to the ICD placement.

Keywords: cardiac amyloidosis; implantable cardioverter-defibrillator; sudden cardiac death; electrophysiological study mapping

1. Introduction

We present a patient with cardiac amyloidosis (CA) resulting from clonal production of immunoglobulin light chains (AL amyloidosis), with recurrent syncope and non-sustained ventricular tachycardia (nsVT), who underwent electrophysiological study with endocardial electro-anatomic voltage mapping, and was finally referred for implantable cardioverter-defibrillator (ICD) placement for primary prevention of sudden cardiac death (SCD).

Two main types of CA are: immunoglobulin light chain (AL) amyloidosis (AL-CA) and transthyretin (ATTR) CA. There has been a steady increase in the diagnosis of CA over the past decade. This is largely due to the development of non-invasive imaging modalities, such as strain echocardiography and scintigraphic nuclear imaging. The prevalence of AL-CA is 8–12 per million per year and it accounts for almost 70% of all newly diagnosed patients with CA [1].

The prognosis in CA is poor, patients typically show symptoms and signs of progressive heart failure. Cardiac arrhythmias, particularly atrial fibrillation are well-documented, but there is less data on ventricular arrhythmias. It has been reported that SCD accounts for up to 50% of all cardiac-related deaths in CA patients [2]. However, a study of AL-CA patients with implanted cardiac rhythm recorder revealed bradycardia with subsequent pulseless electrical activity (PEA) as a terminal rhythm in 62% of deaths [3]. Among 272 loop recordings, only one nsVT was found.

Therefore, the role of ICDs in the primary prevention of SCD in patients with CA is still controversial. On the one hand, there is an increased risk of SCD in CA patients, but other studies do not confirm that they benefit from ICD. It has been most frequently reported in the literature that, despite fairly frequent adequate interventions, ICD therapy does not provide a survival benefit in this patient group. Ventricular arrhythmias can be

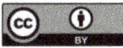

life-threatening, but these are the electromechanical disruptions or conduction disturbances that are considered the most common causes of SCD in patients with CA.

Thus, the role of ICD is uncertain and there are no clear guidelines for such treatment in CA patients. To date, several factors (including cardiac biomarkers and renal function parameters) have been documented to predict overall mortality. However, little is known about risk factors for the arrhythmic cause of SCD in CA patients. Furthermore, little is known about the pathophysiology of ventricular arrhythmias in CA patients, including invasive electrophysiological studies, which is essential for risk assessment [2].

In the presented patient, the endocardial voltage mapping was performed for the first time, which may be important for understanding the causes of arrhythmias in these patients.

2. History of Presentation

A 51-year-old Caucasian male was admitted to the cardiology department for syncope episodes and nsVT recorded on 7-day ambulatory Holter electrocardiographic (ECG) monitoring. On admission, the patient presented with symptoms of heart failure of class II according to the New York Heart Association (NYHA) classification, and occasional chest pain during strenuous exercise. He reported three episodes of syncope during normal activity in the last four months, the course of which could suggest arrhythmias or orthostatic hypotension. Pulse rate was 68 bpm with a regular rhythm, systemic blood pressure 108/69 mm·Hg, a third heart sound was audible on auscultation, but there were no signs of lung congestion or peripheral edema. The medications the patient was taking were diuretics (furosemidum 2 × 40 mg daily, spironolactone 50 mg daily) and ramipril 5 mg daily. The latter was withdrawn on admission due to low BP.

2.1. Past Medical History

Fifteen months earlier this patient was diagnosed with multiple myeloma and concomitant renal and CA resulting from AL fibrils deposit composed of monoclonal immunoglobulin lambda-type light chains (AL amyloidosis). The abdominal fat tissue biopsy revealed amyloid deposits after Congo red staining. Transthoracic echocardiography (TTE) showed biatrial enlargement, concentric left ventricular (LV) and right ventricular (RV) myocardial hypertrophy, preserved LV ejection fraction (LVEF) of 55%, and LV diastolic dysfunction. Cardiac magnetic resonance imaging (cMRI) revealed a spectrum of typical features of CA. The patient was referred for chemotherapy and underwent four cycles according to the MPV regimen (melphalan, prednisone, bortezomib), and later the treatment was changed to VCD (bortezomib, cyclophosphamide, dexamethasone). After one year of treatment, based on the haematological response criteria, a good partial response was obtained (free light chain normalization, significant reduction of proteinuria).

2.2. Investigations

Upon admission blood tests revealed an increased N-terminal pro-brain natriuretic peptide (NT-proBNP) level of 1700 pg/mL (normal: <40 pg/mL) and hs-cTnI concentration of 0.134 ng/mL (normal: <0.034 ng/mL), creatinine level was 1.08 and eGFR 79 mL/min/1.73 m^2 and electrolyte levels were normal. The patient was classified in stage III according to the Mayo 2004 staging system [4]. ECG showed sinus rhythm with low voltage QRS complexes in limb leads, right axis deviation and right bundle branch block. There was no narrowing of coronary arteries in coronary computed tomography angiography, and the Agatston score was 0. Seven-day ambulatory Holter ECG monitoring revealed three nsVT episodes with two different morphologies (the fastest of 169 bpm, and the longest of 7 s and including 20 beats). During Holter monitoring, the patient reported dizziness and worsening of exercise intolerance. TTE demonstrated, as previously, enlargement of the left (36 mL/m^2) and right atrium (28 cm^2), LV hypertrophy (interventricular septum up to 14 mm), mildly reduced LVEF of 50%, a restrictive filling pattern and a significantly abnormal LV global longitudinal strain (GLS) of −10.4% with an apical sparing pattern (Figure 1A,B).

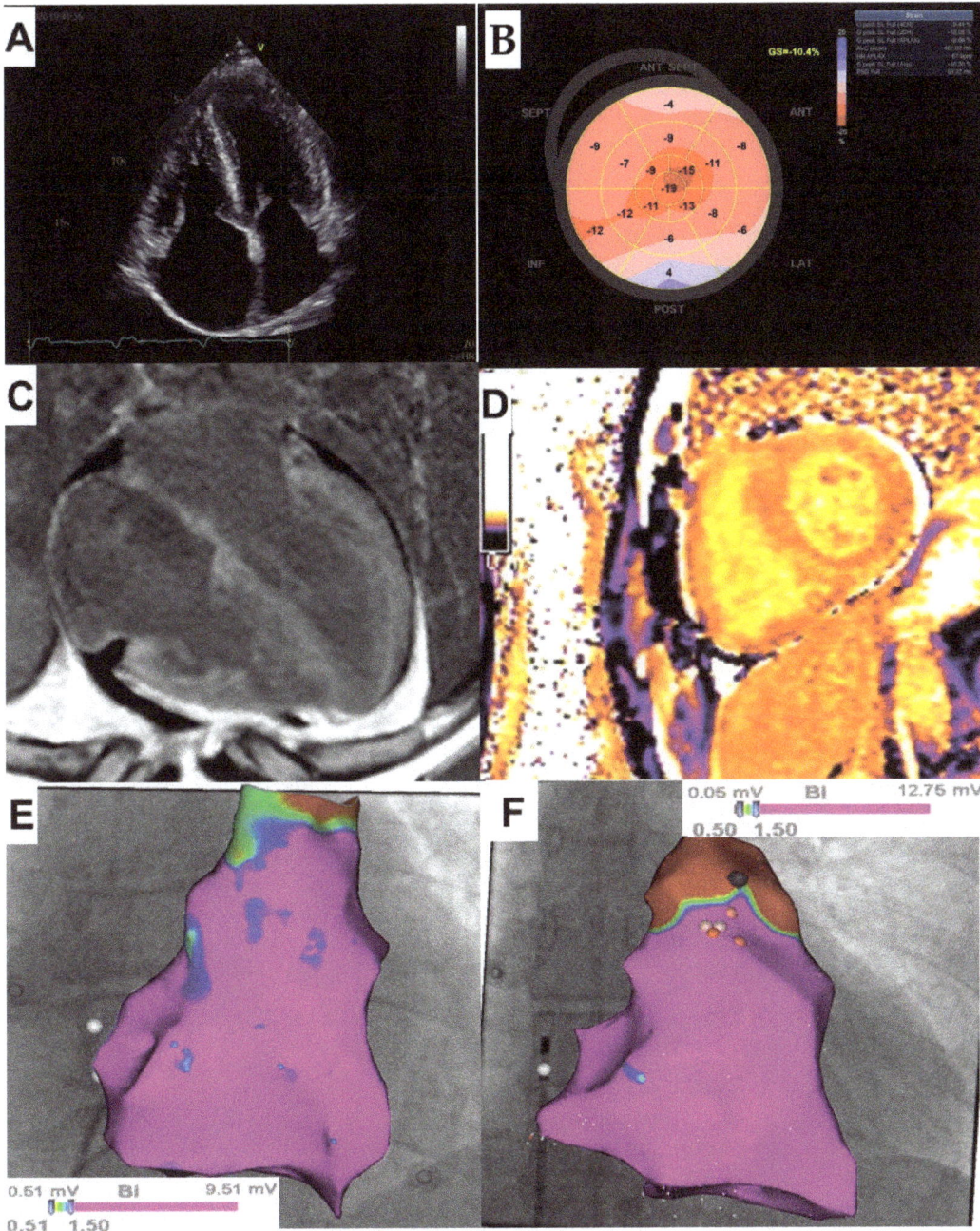

Figure 1. (**A**) Transthoracic echocardiography (TTE Vivid S95, GE Healthcare, Chicago, IL, USA): 4- chamber apical view demonstrating ventricular hypertrophy and atrial enlargement; (**B**) TTE (Vivid S95, GE Healthcare, Chicago, IL, USA): Left ventricular (LV) global longitudinal strain showing LV "apical sparing" pattern; (**C**) Cardiac magnetic resonance imaging (cMRI; Siemens Aera, 1.5 T, Erlangen, Germany): Phase-sensitive inversion recovery sequence showing the extent and distribution

of late gadolinium enhancement (LGE) in the 4-chamber plane. Generalized, diffuse LGE is shown, involving the entire left and right ventricles as well as atrial walls; (**D**) cMRI (Siemens Aera, 1.5 T, Erlangen, Germany): Modified Look-Locker inversion recovery (MOLLI) sequence showing very low post-contrast T1 values, similar to the blood pool values, corresponding to the markedly increased myocardial extracellular volume (ECV) of 70% (reference range: 26 ± 3%); (**E,F**) Bipolar endocardial voltage map of the right ventricle (RV) (3D electroanatomical system CARTO 3, ThermoCool SmartTouch catheter -Biosense Webster Inc, Irvine, CA, USA) obtained in the presented patient with AL cardiac amyloidosis (**E**), and in the patient without any heart disease (**F**). Both patients exhibit normal myocardial bipolar voltages as indicated by a purple color representing normal myocardium with a voltage > 1.5 mV.

The cMRI showed very high native T_1 and T_2 relaxation times, markedly increased extracellular volume fraction (ECV) of 70% and generalized transmural late gadolinium enhancement (LGE) involving the entire LV and RV myocardium as well as the atrial walls (Figure 1C,D). Microvolt T-wave alternans (MTWA) testing was performed on a treadmill, and the result was negative. After approval by a local ethics committee and the patient's written informed consent was obtained (ethical approval reference number: NKBBN/725/2020), an invasive electrophysiology study (EPS) was performed and revealed abnormal sinoatrial and atrioventricular (AV) conduction. The corrected sinus node recovery time (cSNRT) was significantly abnormal: with the first pause at 4.6 s and the second pause at 5.5 s (normal value < 1.5 s). The His bundle-ventricular (HV) interval was prolonged to 62 ms (normal range 35–55 ms). Programmed ventricular stimulation was performed in accordance with the local protocol: up to three extrastimuli at two paced cycle lengths: 600 ms and 400 ms and the pacing site was the RV apex. No arrhythmia was induced. Then, bipolar endocardial electro-anatomic voltage mapping of RV and right atrium was performed with the use of ThermoCool SmartTouch catheter (Biosense Webster Inc., Irvine, CA, USA) and 3D electroanatomical system CARTO 3. It revealed normal voltage of endocardial potentials and no low voltage areas were recorded (Figure 1E). This image was similar to that of a patient without any heart disease, who had intracardiac right heart mapping prior to ablation for ventricular arrhythmia originated from the RV outflow tract (Figure 1F).

Finally, a dual-chamber ICD was inserted (Rivacor 5 DR-T, Biotronik, Germany). During the 12-month follow-up, there were no episodes of arrhythmia in the routine ICD controls.

Currently, the patient is after an autologous stem-cell transplant.

3. Discussion

Among patients with CA, SCD accounts for up to 50% of all cardiac deaths [5]. However, the frequency of arrhythmic SCD is unknown, and electromechanical dissociation or (less commonly) AV conduction disturbances are considered the most common cause of SCD in CA patients. nsVT is commonly found in patients with CA, but has a low predictive value as a risk factor for malignant ventricular arrhythmias [2]. Consequently, the role of ICD is controversial in this group of patients and there are currently no European guidelines on ICD treatment for primary prevention in patients with CA. According to the 2019 Heart Rhythm Society consensus statement, a prophylactic ICD implantation may be considered in patients with AL cardiac amyloidosis and nsVT in whom the expected survival is longer than 1 year [6]. However, this is only a class IIb recommendation. Furthermore, a syncope is a common finding in CA patients, but is a non-specific symptom and may result from various causes, not only arrhythmias, such as orthostatic hypotension, autonomic dysfunction, the use of diuretics or vasodilating drugs, and AV conduction disturbances [2].

In the presented patient, EPS was performed in order to further stratify the risk of SCD. It should be emphasized that EPS is rarely performed in CA patients, and we found only two studies reporting electrophysiological abnormalities among CA patients in EPS. So far, there are no studies that have performed intracardiac mapping in this patient group. Reisinger at al. [5] indicated that markedly prolonged HV interval ($\geq$80 ms) in patients with CA was the only independent predictor for SCD; however, this did not occur in the presented case (HV interval of 62 ms). The HV interval > 55 ms is frequently found in CA patients [2,5]. Its significant prolongation (≥80 ms) may indicate, on the one hand, a risk of complete AV block occurrence due to amyloid infiltration of the conduction system, and on the other hand, a significant infiltration of the myocardium by amyloid fibrils and thus an increased risk of death due to electromechanical dissociation or ventricular arrhythmias [5]. However, ventricular tachyarrhythmias are rarely induced in EPS in CA patients [2,5] and also have not been induced in the presented patient. In turn, low-voltage areas detected during endocardial electro-anatomical mapping may indicate the presence of potential arrhythmogenic substrate for ventricular tachycardia (VT) [7]. However, to our surprise, the results of right heart voltage mapping our patient did not reveal any abnormalities, suggesting that the substrate for VT (if any) may be difficult to identify. Additionally, we found no correlation between the electro-anatomical mapping (absence of low voltage areas in the right heart) and LGE (diffuse, involving most of the myocardium). Furthermore, the MTWA testing, which was previously considered a predictor of increased risk of SCD in patients with heart failure, was negative in the presented case [8]. Nevertheless, based on the current knowledge and the proposed algorithm (Figure 2), the final decision was to implant an ICD. The patient reported recurrent syncope, nsVT was documented, but was in a relatively early stage of heart disease as indicated by the mildly elevated cardiac biomarkers and preserved LVEF. However, the patient was diagnosed with reduced LV GLS and diffuse transmural LGE, which are considered markers potentially identifying CA patients that may benefit from ICD implantation [2].

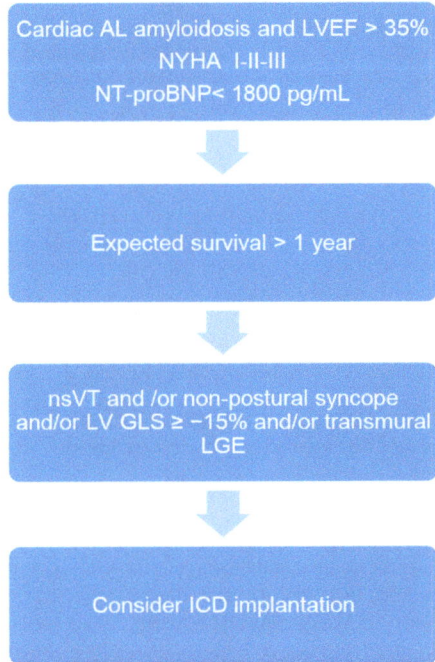

Figure 2. The algorithm proposed for qualifying cardiac immunoglobulin-derived light chains amyloidosis (AL) patients for ICD implantation in primary prevention of sudden cardiac death (2). ICD: implantable cardioverter-defibrillator; LVEF: left ventricular ejection fraction; NT-proBNP: N-terminal pro brain natriuretic peptide; nsVT: non-sustained ventricular tachycardia; LV GLS: left ventricular global longitudinal strain; LGE: late gadolinium enhancement.

On the other hand, there were no abnormalities in endocardial voltage mapping of RV and right atrium, and supposing that in AL amyloidosis, amyloid fibrils infiltrate both left and right ventricles, it can be assumed that the result of LV endocardial mapping would be similar. The significance of these findings is evidenced by the fact that during the 12-month follow-up, the patient did not develop any ventricular arrhythmias. However, the occurrence of arrhythmias with a slower rate than the programmed detection rate of the ICD cannot be excluded. This could potentially cause an underestimation of arrhythmia burden. Therefore, EPS testing may be considered to better stratify the risk of SCD in patients with CA and nsVT.

4. Conclusions

Data on the role of EPS in CA patients are limited. Normal voltage of endocardial potentials, found for the first time in a patient with AL amyloidosis, in combination with a negative result of programmed ventricular stimulation, may indicate a small potential arrhythmogenic substrate in patients with CA. This is in line with the observation that patients with CA do not benefit from ICD for primary prevention. Further prospective studies are needed to understand the pathophysiology of arrhythmias in CA patients and thus to better stratify the risk of arrhythmic SCD.

Author Contributions: Conceptualization, E.L., M.K., A.L-S.; investigation, T.K., K.D.; writing—original draft preparation, A.L.-S.; writing—review and editing, E.L., A.D.-K.; visualization, G.S.; supervision, E.L., T.K.; All authors have read and agreed to the published version of the manuscript.

Funding: This research was completed without external funding.

Institutional Review Board Statement: The study was conducted according to the guidelines of the Declaration of Helsinki, and approved by the Independent Bioethics Committee for Scientific Research at Medical University of Gdansk– NKBBN/725/2020.

Informed Consent Statement: Written informed consent has been obtained from the patient to publish this paper.

Data Availability Statement: Not applicable.

Conflicts of Interest: The authors declare no conflict of interest.

References

1. Oerlemans, M.I.F.J.; Rutten, K.H.G.; Minnema, M.C.; Raymakers, R.A.P.; Asselbergs, F.W.; de Jonge, N. Cardiac amyloidosis: The need for early diagnosis. *Neth. Heart J.* **2019**, *27*, 525–536. [CrossRef]
2. Liżewska-Springer, A.; Sławiński, G.; Lewicka, E. Arrhythmic Sudden Cardiac Death and the Role of Implantable Cardioverter-Defibrillator in Patients with Cardiac Amyloidosis-A Narrative Literature Review. *J. Clin. Med.* **2021**, *10*, 1858. [CrossRef] [PubMed]
3. Sayed, R.H.; Rogers, D.; Khan, F.; Wechalekar, A.D.; Lachmann, H.J.; Fontana, M.; Mahmood, S.; Sachchithanantham, S.; Patel, K.; Hawkins, P.N.; et al. A study of implanted cardiac rhythm recorders in advanced cardiac AL amyloidosis. *Eur. Heart J.* **2015**, *7*, 1098–1105. [CrossRef] [PubMed]
4. Dispenzieri, A.; Gertz, M.A.; Kyle, R.A.; Lacy, M.Q.; Burritt, M.F.; Therneau, T.M.; Greipp, P.R.; Witzig, T.E.; Lust, J.A.; Rajkumar, S.V.; et al. Serum cardiac troponins and N-terminal pro-brain natriuretic peptide: A staging system for primary systemic amyloidosis. *J. Clin. Oncol.* **2004**, *22*, 3751–3757. [CrossRef] [PubMed]
5. Reisinger, J.; Dubrey, S.W.; Lavalley, M.; Skinner, M.; Falk, R.H. Electrophysiologic abnormalities in AL (primary) amyloidosis with cardiac involvement. *J. Am. Coll. Cardiol.* **1997**, *30*, 1046–1051. [CrossRef]
6. Towbin, J.A.; McKenna, W.J.; Abrams, D.J.; Ackerman, M.J.; Calkins, H.; Darrieux, F.C.C.; Daubert, J.P.; de Chillou, C.; DePasquale, E.C.; Desai, M.Y.; et al. 2019 HRS expert consensus statement on evaluation, risk stratification, and management of arrhythmogenic cardiomyopathy. *Heart Rhythm.* **2019**, *16*, e301–e372. [CrossRef] [PubMed]
7. Letsas, K.P.; Efremidis, M.; Vlachos, K.; Asvestas, D.; Takigawa, M.; Bazoukis, G.; Frontera, A.; Giannopoulos, G.; Saplaouras, A.; Sakellaropoulou, A.; et al. Right ventricular outflow tract low-voltage areas identify the site of origin of idiopathic ventricular arrhythmias: A high-density mapping study. *J. Cardiovasc. Electrophysiol.* **2019**, *30*, 2362–2369. [CrossRef] [PubMed]
8. Merchant, F.M.; Sayadi, O.; Moazzami, K.; Puppala, D.; Armoundas, A.A. T-wave alternans as an arrhythmic risk stratifier: State of the art. *Curr. Cardiol. Rep.* **2013**, *15*, 398. [CrossRef] [PubMed]

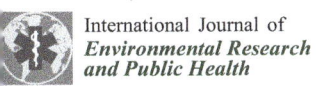

Article

A Study of Major and Minor Complications of 1500 Transvenous Lead Extraction Procedures Performed with Optimal Safety at Two High-Volume Referral Centers

Łukasz Tułecki [1], Anna Polewczyk [2,3,*], Wojciech Jacheć [4], Dorota Nowosielecka [1], Konrad Tomków [1], Paweł Stefańczyk [1], Jarosław Kosior [5], Krzysztof Duda [5], Maciej Polewczyk [6,7] and Andrzej Kutarski [8]

1. Department of Cardiac Surgery, The Pope John Paul II Province Hospital of Zamość, 22-400 Zamość, Poland; luke27@poczta.onet.pl (Ł.T.); dornowos@wp.pl (D.N.); konradtomkow@wp.pl (K.T.); paolost@interia.pl (P.S.)
2. Department of Physiology Pathophysiology and Clinical Immunology, Collegium Medicum, The Jan Kochanowski University, 25-317 Kielce, Poland
3. Department of Cardiac Surgery, Świętokrzyskie Cardiology Center, 25-736 Kielce, Poland
4. 2nd Department of Cardiology, Silesian Medical University, 41-808 Zabrze, Poland; wjachec@interia.pl
5. Department of Cardiology, Masovian Specialist Hospital of Radom, 26-617 Radom, Poland; jaroslaw.kosior@icloud.com (J.K.); kadeder@gmail.com (K.D.)
6. Department of Microbiology, Collegium Medicum, Jan Kochanowski Univeristy, 25-369 Kielce, Poland; Maciek.polewczyk@gmail.com
7. Intensive Care Unit, Świętokrzyskie Cardiology Center, 25-736 Kielce, Poland
8. Department of Cardiology, Medical University, 20-059 Lublin, Poland; a_kutarski@yahoo.com
* Correspondence: annapolewczyk@wp.pl

Abstract: *Background:* Transvenous lead extraction (TLE) is the preferred management strategy for complications related to cardiac implantable electronic devices. TLE sometimes can cause serious complications. *Methods:* Outcomes of TLE procedures using non-powered mechanical sheaths were analyzed in 1500 patients (mean age 68.11 years; 39.86% females) admitted to two high-volume centers. *Results:* Complete procedural success was achieved in 96.13% of patients; clinical success in 98.93%, no periprocedural death occurred. Mean lead dwell time in the study population was 112.1 months. Minor complications developed in 115 (7.65%), major complications in 33 (2.20%) patients. The most frequent minor complications were tricuspid valve damage (TVD) (3.20%) and pericardial effusion that did not necessitate immediate intervention (1.33%). The most common major complication was cardiac laceration/vascular tear (1.40%) followed by an increase in TVD by two or three grades to grade 4 (0.80%). *Conclusions:* Despite the long implant duration (112.1 months) satisfying results without procedure-related death can be obtained using mechanical tools. Lead remnants or severe tricuspid regurgitation was the principal cause of lack of clinical and procedural success. Worsening TR(Tricuspid regurgitation) (due to its long-term consequences), but not cardiac/vascular wall damage; is still the biggest TLE-related problem; when non-powered mechanical sheaths are used as first-line tools.

Keywords: transvenous lead extraction; minor and major complications; cardiac laceration/vascular tear; epicardial fluid; tricuspid valve damage

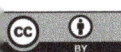

1. Introduction

Transvenous lead extraction (TLE) is considered an integral part of the management strategy for complications related to the presence of cardiac implantable electronic devices (CIED) [1–5].Due to the foreign body reaction and extensive fibrotic scarring around the leads [6,7], TLE can sometimes cause severe damage to the veins and heart as manifested by bleeding into the mediastinum or right pleural cavity, or acute pericardial effusion depending on the location of the tear [1–5,8–12].Another problem we face in TLE is the real risk of tricuspid valve damage (TVD) with worsening tricuspid regurgitation (TR).

The problem of TVD was omitted in the older guidelines [1–4] and addressed only just in the recent ones [4,5]. There are several reports concerning the role of cardiac surgery and cardiac anesthesiology in the management TLE-related cardiovascular injuries [8–12] and TLE effectiveness [13–18], but there is no comprehensive investigation of cardiac laceration/vascular walltear (CVWT) and TVD as major and minor complications of lead extraction. Some investigators reported TR increase without any reference to minor and major TLE complication [19–25]. At our center all cases of symptomatic cardiac tamponade were managed with sternotomy, therefore we were able to provide more precise information about the location of tears. Additionally, continuous TEE (Trans esophageal echocardiography) monitoring enabled a more rapid and accurate assessment of worsening TR.

The aim of the present study was to determine the occurrence and describe in detail cardiac/vascular wall rupture and TV damage as a form of major and minor complications related to TLE. Particular attention was paid to the worsening of tricuspid regurgitation and the difficulty in classification.

2. Material and Methods

2.1. Study Population

This study was a post hoc analysis of the clinical data of 1500 patients undergoing transvenous lead extraction at two high-volume TLE centers between June 2015 and April 2021. All extraction procedures were performed by the same first operator and nurses in compliance with the same optimal safety regulations. All information relating to patients and procedures was entered into a computer on an ongoing basis. Conventional mechanical sheaths were the first-line tools; powered rotational mechanical sheaths and other instruments were used as the second option. Laser sheaths were not used at our centers.

2.2. Lead Extraction Procedure

Lead extraction procedures were defined according to the most recent guidelines on the management of lead-related complications (HRS 2017 and EHRA 2018) [4,5]. Indications for TLE and type of periprocedural complications were defined according to the 2017 HRS Expert Consensus Statement on Cardiovascular Implantable Electronic Device Lead Management and Extraction [4].

Most removal procedures were performed using non-powered mechanical systems such as polypropylene Byrd dilator sheaths (Cook® Medical, Leechburg, PA, USA), if only possible via the implant vein. If technical difficulties arose, additional tools such as Evolution (Cook® Medical, Leechburg, PA, USA), TightRail (Spectranetix, Colorado Springs, CO, USA), lassos, basket catheters and/or alternative venous approaches were utilized. The excimer laser was not applied.

All TLE procedures were performed following the same organizational model. The operating team consisted of a very experienced TLE operator, cardiac surgeon, anesthesiologist and echocardiographist. The procedures were performed in a hybrid room or an operating room on the cardiac surgery ward, with a full range of equipment for an emergency rescue.

The SAFeTY TLE score was used to assess the risk for the occurrence of major complications related to TLE [26] using an online calculator, available at http://alamay2.linuxpl.info/kalkulator/ (accessed on 11 September 2021).

2.3. TEE Monitoring during TLE

Echocardiography, especially continuous transesophageal echocardiography (TEE) is a very useful tool that improves the safety of TLE procedures [27]. In this study, TEE was performed by two experienced echocardiographers using Philips iE33, GE Vivid S 70 and GE Vivid E-95(GE Vivid S 70 and GE Vivid E-95—both GE Medical Systems, San Francisco, CA, USA) machines equipped with X7-2t Live 3D or 6VT-D probes. All examinations were archived and information was stored in a computer database. The applications of

TEE included preprocedural assessment of lead position with particular emphasis on the presence of additional masses on the leads, evaluation of tricuspid valve function and navigation of lead removal, whereas postoperative TEE was used to determine procedure effectiveness and possible complications [28–30].

Intraoperative TEE allowed visualization of direct pulling on the heart during lead extraction, helping explain a frequent drop in blood pressure due to right ventricular collapse [27–29]. A very important role of TEE is to rapidly detect accumulation of blood in the pericardial sac. If the walls of the heart are damaged, TEE can help locate the perforation site by identifying the segment of the wall on which the greatest pulling force is exerted. Additionally, TEE provides information not only on the volume of blood in the pericardial sac and the diastolic function of the right ventricle, but also on the location of fluid and blood clots in terms of the chances of successful pericardial puncture [28,29]. The postoperative phase of TLE includes the evaluation of tricuspid valve function and the assessment of lead remnants, residual vegetations and free-floating fragments of fibrous encapsulation.

2.4. Management of Symptomatic Cardiac Laceration/Vascular Wall Tear

From the very beginning all TLE procedures in the two hospitals have been performed in compliance with the available recommendations [2–5] in terms of the venue, participation of cardiac surgeons and anesthesia teams, continuous blood pressure monitoring, TEE monitoring and measurements of partial pressure of carbon dioxide in the expired air. The availability of cardiac surgeons with surgical instruments and nursing staff made an attempt at pericardiocentesis unreasonable, therefore the preferred choice was proper surgery without further delay (except one patient with borderline hemodynamic values). With this strategy, all urgent interventions were successful and effective, none of the patients died. Only in 2 out of 21 patients with cardiac laceration/vascular wall tear (CVWT) in our series required the use of cardiopulmonary bypass pump (CPB) to support the circulation. One patient required simultaneous urgent tricuspid valve repair and another one reconstruction of the superior vena cava together with TV repair and replacement. In the remaining 19 patients CPB was not necessary.

2.5. Assessment of Tricuspid Valve Damage

The postprocedural phase of TEE monitoring includes reassessment of cardiac/vascular wall injuries and as exact as possible reevaluation of TV function (including the comparison with baseline findings). The mid-esophageal, inferior esophageal and modified transgastric views were applied to visualize the right heart chambers and the tricuspid valve [30]. For visualization of the entire cardiac anatomy and assessment of the course of the lead non-standard imaging planes were sometimes required. The projections and consecutive stages of echocardiographic monitoring were described in detail in previous publications [27–30].

2.6. Presentation of Study Results

Categorical variables were presented as numbers and percentages, and continuous variables were expressed as the mean and standard deviation (SD)

Approval of the Bioethics Committee

The study was carried out in accordance with the ethical standards of the 1964 Declaration of Helsinki. All patients gave their informed written consent to undergo TLE and to use anonymous data from their medical records, which was approved by the Bioethics Committee at the Regional Chamber of Physicians in Lublin no. 288/2018/KB/VII.

3. Results

The study population consisted of 1500 patients (mean age 68.11 years, 39.86% of women). The mean dwell time of the oldest extracted lead per patient was 112.1 months, the sum of lead dwell times was 17.01 years. The total number of major and minor complications was 33 (2.20%) and 115 (7.67%), respectively. Complete procedural success was obtained in 96.13%, partial radiographic success in 3.07%, whereas clinical success in 98.93% of the 1500 patients/procedures (Table 1).

Table 1. Clinical characteristics of the study population.

Characteristics of the Study Population	Count/Average	%/SD
Patient age at TLE [years]	68.11	14.02
Patient age at first system implantation [years]	58.81	15.77
Sex (% of female patients)	598	39.86%
Etiology: IHD, MI	979	65.27%
Underlying disease: cardiomyopathy, valvular heart disease	277	18.47%
Underlying disease: congenital, channelopathies, neurocardiogenic indications, cardiac surgery	243	16.20%
LVEF average [%]	49.26	15.92
Renal failure: patients with creatinine concentration > 2.00/dL	375	25.00%
Previous sternotomy	214	14.27%
Charlson comorbidity index [points]	5.10	3.76
Systemic infection (with or without pocket infection)	230	15.33%
Local (pocket) infection	90	6.00%
Lead failure (replacement)	865	58.33%
Change of pacing mode/upgrading, downgrading	110	7.33%
Other: Abandoned lead/prevention of abandonment, (AF, redundant leads), threatening/potentially threatening lead (loops, free ending, left heart, LDTD) Other (MRI indications, cancer, painful pocket, loss of indication for pacing/ICD) regainingvenous access (symptomatic occlusion, SVC syndrome, lead replacement/upgrading)	193	12.87%
System: pacemaker (any)	1008	67.08%
System: ICD (VVI, DDD)	359	23.97%
System: CRT-D	133	8.87%
Dwell time of the oldest lead per patient [months]	112.1	78.16
Sum of lead dwell times [years]	17.01	13.75
Major complications	33	2.20%
Minor complications	115	7.66%
Complete procedural success	1442	96.13%
Partial radiographic success	46	3.07%
Clinical success	1484	98.93%

Abbreviations: CRT-D—cardiac resynchronization therapy defibrillator, DDD—dual-chamber antibradycardia pacing, ICD—implantable cardioverter defibrillator, IHD—ischemic heart disease, LDTD—lead-dependent tricuspid dysfunction, LVEF—left ventricular ejection fraction, MI—myocardial infarction, SVC—superior vena cava, TLE—transvenous lead extraction, VVI—ventricular demand pacing.

The most important reason for the absence of clinical and procedural success was the lack of complete procedural success (a non-extractable tip of the lead or lead fragments < 4 cm left behind in the heart). However, even the presence of lead remnants can be regarded as clinically acceptable, if procedure indications are non-infectious. In infectious cases incomplete lead removal is considered as failure to achieve clinical success despite the absence of negative effects on the course of infection. The second reason for no clinical and procedural success was a severe increase in tricuspid regurgitation meeting the echocardiographic criteria for cardiac surgery. Severe deterioration of TV function not necessitating surgery was categorized as minor complications. Despite the need to perform 21 surgical rescue interventions there was no procedure-related death that otherwise would be the reason for no clinical or procedural success. It should be emphasized that contrary to popular opinion, the leading TLE-related problem is still worsening TR (due to its long-term consequences) but not cardiac/vascular wall damage when non-powered mechanical sheaths are used as the first-line option (Table 2).

Table 2. Effectiveness and safety of TLE.

Causes of Clinical Failure	Patients	%
Clinical success	1484	98.93%
Lead tip left behind– infection	4	0.27%
Significant TLE-related TV damage	12	0.80%
Procedure-related death (intra- or postprocedural)	0	0.00%
All patients	1500	100.0%
Causes of procedural failure		
Procedural success	1442	96.13%
Lead tip left behind	16	1.07%
Lead remnant (<4.0 cm)	30	2.00%
Significant TLE-related TV damage	12	0.80%
Procedure-related death (intra-, postprocedural)	0	0.00%
All patients	1500	100.0%

Abbreviations: TLE—transvenous lead extraction, TV—tricuspid valve.

Minor complications after TLE were observed in 115 (7.67%) patients. The most frequent complication was tricuspid valve damage (worsening by two or three degrees but not to grade 4) detected in 43 patients (2.91%). Worsening by one degree only was not considered minor complication because such a difference may be very subtle leading to an error caused for instance by fluid oversupply. Another minor complication in the present study was pericardial effusion not requiring pericardiocentesis or surgical intervention. It was detected in 24 patients (1.60%). Hemodynamic monitoring (TEE, arterial line, breath gas analysis) helped avoid pericardiocentesis despite a transient drop in blood pressure. The third minor complication (1.33%) was blood transfusion related to blood loss during surgery (the need for transfusion of more than one unit of red blood cells). Hematoma at the surgical site requiring drainage (13 patients, 0.87%) and pneumothorax requiring a chest tube (3 patients, 0.20%) or not (1 patient, 0.067%) were less common (Table 3). This study reveals that worsening TR (12 categorized as major complication, 43 as minor complication and 106 not classified as minor complication) remains the biggest challenge in lead extraction technology (Table 3).

Major complications were observed in 33 (2.20%) patients. The rate appears slightly higher than reported by other investigators but one should bear in mind the prolonged lead dwell time per patient (112.1 months) and the sum of lead dwell times (17.01 years) in the present study. The most common major complication in the 33 patients was cardiac laceration/vascular wall tear (22 lesions in 21 patients, 1.40%) followed by severe tricuspid valve damage (by 2 or 3 degrees to grade 4 in 12 patients, 0.80%). Table 4 summarizes the types of cardiac laceration/vascular wall tear (CVWT) in the 21 patients. Right atrial appendage (RAA) rupture (one double) occurred in 8 patients (0.53%), tear of the connection of the right atrium (RA) to the superior vena cava (SVC) in 5 (0.33%) and SVC laceration in 3 patients (0.20%) (in 2 patients caused by a guidewire or a new lead that passed into the right pleura after lead removal). Other injuries were sporadic and included lateral wall tear (double), RA tear and injury to the coronary sinus (CS) ostium and tear of the connection of the RA to the inferior vena cava (IVC), tear of the right ventricular (RV) wall. Summing up, the connection of the SVC to the RA, RAA wall, and the SVC alone was the most common location of CVWT (16 cases out of 21 requiring surgical repair = 76.19%) but the ventricular wall was affected only in 4.8% of all CVWTs (Table 4).

Table 3. Analysis of minor complications.

Minor Complications	Patients	%
Number of minor complications	115	7.67%
Tricuspid valve damage by 2 degrees but not to grade 4	43	2.91%
Pericardial effusion not requiring pericardiocentesis or surgical intervention	20	1.33%
Blood transfusion related to blood loss during surgery	17	1.13%
Hematoma at the surgical site requiring drainage	13	0.87%
Arm swelling or lead-induced venous thrombosis resulting in medical intervention	4	0.29%
Pneumothorax requiring a chest tube	3	0.20%
Blood transfusion related to blood loss during surgery	1	0.067%
Arm swelling or lead-induced venous thrombosis	1	0.067%
Tricuspid valve damage + pericardial effusion not requiring pericardiocentesis	1	0.067%
Tricuspid valve damage + hemothorax not requiring a chest tube	1	0.067%
Pericardial effusion + pneumothorax not requiring intervention	1	0.067%
Pericardial effusion not requiring pericardiocentesis + blood transfusion	1	0.067%
Pericardial effusion not requiring pericardiocentesis + vascular repair at lead venous entry site + blood transfusion	1	0.067%
Migrated lead fragment without sequelae	1	0.067%
Femoral vein thrombosis	1	0.067%
Other mixed	5	0.34%
All patients	1500	100.000%

Table 4. Analysis of major complications.

Major Complications	Patients	%
Number of major complications	33	2.20%
Hemopericardium:rescue cardiac surgery	17	1.13%
Hemopericardium drainage (pericardiocentesis)	1	0.067%
Hemothorax:rescue cardiac surgery	2	0.13%
Acute heart failure (decrease in BP and contractility as a reaction to guide wire in mediastinum)	1	0.067%
Severe tricuspid valve damage (by 2 or 3 degrees to grade 4)	11	0.733%
Double (hemopericardium rescue cardiac surgery, tricuspidvalve damage)	1	0.067%
All patients	1500	100.0%
Types of cardiovascular damage in 21 patients		
RAA wall tear (one double)	8	0.53%
Tear of connection of RA to SVC	5	0.33%
Tear of VCS (in 2 symptoms occurred after lead removal and when guide wire or new lead passed to right pleura)	3	0.20%
Rupture of connection of RAA to RV (partial RAA rupture)	1	0.067%
Tear of lateral wall (double)	1	0.067%
Tear of RA and CS	1	0.067%
Tear of connection of RA to IVC	1	0.067%
Tear of RV	1	0.067%
All patients requiring surgical intervention (one pericardiocentesis only)	21	100.0%

Abbreviations: BP—blood pressure, CS—coronary sinus, IVC—inferior vena cava, RA—right atrium, RAA—right atrial appendage, RV—right ventricle, SVC—superior venacava.

Table 5 provides a succinct description of the TEE findings that preceded the buildup of pericardial fluid, i.e., blood pooling around the heart, changes in arterial blood pressure and CO^2 in exhaled air since the onset of CVWT to the cessation of bleeding.

Table 5. Description of the symptoms of cardiac and vascular damage during TLE.

Clinical Course and Hemodynamic Changes since Symptom Onset to Bleeding Cessation	Number of Patients	Max Drop in Blood Pressure [mmHg]	Max HR Change [per minute]	Max Decrease in CO_2 [mmHg]	Global Loss of Blood Volume [mL]
RAA wall tear (one double)	8	52.82 ± 25.13	6.15 ± 13.81	3.82 ± 2.82	1628.8 ± 2164.8
Rupture of connection of RAA to RV (partial RAA rupture)	1	30	5	5	800
Tear of connection of RA to SVC	5	53.73 ± 25.92	18.32 ± 7.62	7.01 ± 2.03	2200.0 ± 1881.4
Tear of lateral wall: double	1	70	−20	1	1500
Tear of RA and CS wall	1	55	10	5	5000
Tear of connection of RA to IVC	1	73	0	3	600
Tear of SVC wall (in 2 cases after lead removal and when a guide wire or new lead passed to the right pleura)	3	65.33 ± 27.23	10.32 ± 3.37	4.12 ± 3.27	3200.4 ± 1453.2
Tear of RV wall	1	75	0	6	1100

Abbreviations: BP—blood pressure, CS—coronary sinus, HR—heart rate, IVC—inferior vena cava, RA—right atrium, RAA—right atrial appendage, RV—right ventricle, SVC—superior vena cava.

The amount of pericardial fluid depends mainly on the size of the rupture but the rapidity with which the bleeding may be stopped depends on the location of the tear. The present study shows that an injury to structures other than the RA (CS, SVC, connection of RA to IVC) was associated with a higher drop in arterial blood pressure and CO^2 in exhaled air and a much higher blood loss (blood volume drained during rescue operation) than in cardiac tamponade caused by RA damage. All these findings confirm the differences in the clinical manifestations between damage to the RA and injury to other structures, which seem to be more serious and difficult to manage (Table 5).

The less frequently addressed problem is TLE-related TV damage. Worsening TR is a common term for a wide spectrum of echocardiographic images [19–25]. This procedure-related TV damage is often superimposed on the previously existing TV dysfunction and it may be difficult to discern the new from the old. The role of an echocardiographer is relatively simple: to describe as exactly as possible TV function and changes from baseline. However, physicians generating inputs to medical databases and preparing discharge summaries may face the problem of how to categorize the worsening of TR: as a non-significant phenomenon (the borderline diagnosis)? minor complication? or major complication? All major complications have to be discussed with the cardiac surgeon regarding the TV replacement.

In the present study, mild TR (grade 1) wasa very frequent finding (49.43% of patients) prior to TLE. Moderate (grade 2), intermediate (grade 3) and severe (grade 4) forms of TR were less common (21.75%, 17.24% and 7.68%, respectively). Changes in the severity of regurgitation after TLE included both an increase (in 10.09% of patients) and a decrease in TR (in 10.30% of patients). The most common finding about TV function after TLE was either worsening or improvement by one degree. It may indicate that the differences by one degree (both directions) are very subtle and are not only "examiner-dependent" but also condition-dependent (rapid fluid intake). On the other hand worsening from grade 3 to grade 4 may have clinical consequences. Lead-dependent TV dysfunction (LDTD) was not the subject of this paper so we did not tackle the issue. Rupture of the chordae tendineae was an additional finding which was observed in moderate and severe TV worsening (43 patients, 2.91%). A moderate increase in TR by 2 or 3 degrees, but not to grade 4 (31 patients 2.10%) was considered minor complication and a significant increase in TR by 2 degrees to grade 4 was considered major complication (Table 6).

Table 6. Analysis of tricuspid valve function before and after TLE.

Tricuspid Regurgitation Before TLE		
Degree of tricuspid regurgitation	No. of patients	%
Lack (grade 0)	58	3.91%
Mild (grade 1)	734	49.43%
Moderate (grade 2)	323	21.75%
Intermediate (grade 3)	256	17.24%
Severe (grade 4)	114	7.68%
All	1485	100.0%
Lack of examination, not described	15	
Mild (0,1)	792	53.33%
Moderate/intermediate (2,3)	579	38.99%
Severe (4)	114	7.68%
All	1485	100.0%
Lack of examination, not described	15	
Changes in TR after TLE		
Direction of changes in TR	No. of patients	%
No changes	1175	79.61%
Increase by 1 degree	106	7.18%
Increase by 2 degrees	35	2.37%
Increase by 3 degrees	8	0.542%
Decrease by 1 degree	131	8.87%
Decrease by 2 degrees	21	1.42%
All examined patients	1476	100.0%
Lack of examination, not described	24	
Worsening tricuspid regurgitation after TLE		
	No. of patients	%
Rupture of chordae tendineae	47	3.18%
Moderate increase in TR by 2 or 3 degree but not to grade 4	31	2.10%
Significant (by 2 degrees) increase in TR to grade 4	12	0.813%
Management of TV damage as TLE major complication	No. of patients	% among 12 (% among 1500)
TV replacement (2 acute, 3 late)	5	41.67% (0.33%)
Classified as refused operation but general condition unchanged	3	25.00% (0.20%)
Not classified, remained under observation	3	25.00% (0.20%)
Disqualification—cancer disease	1	8.33% (0.067%)
All	12	100.0%

Abbreviations: TLE—transvenous lead extraction, TR—tricuspid regurgitation, TV—tricuspid valve.

In 12 patients worsening TR was classified as major complication. TV replacement (2 acute, 3 late) was performed in 5 patients (41.67% out of 12 i.e., 0.33% out of 1500). Three patients were not classified (slight improvement in control TTE examination) and remained under observation (25.00% out of 12, 0.20% out of 1500). The same number of patients refused TV replacement and they also remained under observation (Table 6).

Table 7 summarizes the occurrence of worsening TR as no complication, minor or major complication after TLE. The data suggests that the worsening of TR by one degree to grade 1 and 2 may be disregarded as a complication. The worsening of TR by one degree from grade 2 to 3 and from grade 3 to 4 remains controversial. Such worsening may be symptomatic.

Table 7. Classification of tricuspid regurgitation after TLE.

Worsening TR after TLE	Number of Patients	TR before TLE	TR after TLE	% (n = 149)	% (n = 1476)	Present Classification	Suggested Classification
Increase by 1 degree	27	0	1	18.12%	1.83%	Lack	Lack
	38	1	2	25.50%	2.57%	Lack	Lack
	25	2	3	16.78%	1.69%	Lack	Minor
	16	3	4	10.74%	1.08%	Lack	Minor
Increase by 2 degrees	1	0	2	0.671%	0.067%	Minor	Minor
	30	1	3	20.13%	2.10%	Minor	Minor
	4	2	4	2.68%	0.27%	Major	Major
Increase by 3 degrees	8	1	4	5.37%	0.54%	Major	Major
All (n, %)	149			100.0%			

Lack—lack of complication, Minor—minor complication, Major—major complication.

4. Discussion

Transvenous lead extraction is an integral part of the management of CIED-related problems [1–5]. Cardiac and venous injuries during lead extraction are complications with potentially serious consequences. So far there has been no in-depth analysis that would go beyond injury to the SVC/other vessels and attempt to identify TLE-related TV damage (TVD) as minor and major complications of lead extraction.

Despite the long implant duration major complications occurred in 33 out of 1500 (2.20%) patients, whereas minor complications in 115 (7.67%) patients. Complete procedural success was obtained in 96.13%, partial radiographic success in 3.07%, clinical success in 98.93% of 1500 patients/procedures. The most important reason for the absence of clinical and procedural success was the lack of complete radiographic success. The second reason was severe worsening of tricuspid regurgitation meeting echocardiographic criteria for cardiac surgery. Marked deterioration in TV function but not requiring surgery was classified as minor complication. Despite the need for rescue surgery in 21 cases there was no procedure-related death that otherwise would account for the lack of clinical or procedural success. Tricuspid valve damage was the most common minor complication (3.07%). The second minor complication was pericardial effusion not requiring pericardiocentesis or surgical intervention (1.60%). Less frequent minor complications included blood transfusion related to blood loss during surgery (1.33%), hematoma at the surgical site requiring drainage (0.87%) and pneumothorax requiring a chest tube (0.20%) or not (0.067%). Major complications occurred in 2.20% of cases but one should bear in mind that the dwell time of the oldest lead per patient was 112.1 months. The most common major complication was cardiac laceration/vascular wall tear (1.47%) followed by severe tricuspid valve damage (0.80%). The most frequent location of the tear was RAA (0.53%), connection of RA to SVC (0.33%) and SVC (0.20%). Other locations were rare (lateral RA, CS ostium, connection of RA to IVC). There was only one rupture of RVA wall. An injury to structures other than RA (CS, SVC, connection of RA to IVC) was associated with higher drops in arterial blood pressure and CO_2 in exhaled air and much higher blood losses (blood volume drained during rescue operation) than in tamponade caused by RA damage.

All these findings confirm the differences in the clinical manifestations between damage to the RA and injury to other structures, which seem to be more serious and difficult to manage. The worsening of TR related to TLE is a common term for a wide spectrum of echocardiographic images. TR after TLE can either worsen (10.09%) or improve (10.30%). The most frequent finding was worsening or improvement by one degree. Rupture of chordae tendineae was detected as an additional finding in moderate and severe TR worsening (3.21%). Moderate increases in TR by 2 degrees, but not to grade 4 (2.37%) were considered minor complications and significant (by 2 degrees) increase in TR but to grade 4 was considered major complication. In 12 patients worsening TR was classified as major complication. TV replacement was performed (2 acute, 3 late) in 5 patients (41.67% among 12), 3 pts were not selected for surgery (slight improvement in control TTE examinations) and remained under observation. The same number of patients refused TV replacement and they also remained under observation. In terms of classification as lack, minor or major complication after TLE this study suggests that the worsening of TR after TLE by one degree from grade 1 and 2 may be disregarded as a complication. The worsening of TR by one degree from grade 2 to 3 and from grade 3 to 4 remains controversial. Once again, contrary to popular opinion, the leading TLE-related problem is still worsening TR (due to its long-term consequences) but not cardiac/vascular wall damage when non-powered mechanical sheaths are used as the first-line tools.

If excimer laser energy is not applied, major complications other than tear of the SVC and anonymous vein seem to be more frequent [18]. The available guidelines and medical literature describe all forms of cardiovascular wall tear but not worsening TR after TLE [1–5,16–18].

There are two large reports concerning vascular and cardiac wall damage during lead extraction using laser technique. Brunner et al. found out that the rate of complications requiring rescue intervention was 0.8% (mean implant duration time 4.9 years in overall cohort). SVC laceration was most frequent (80%), whereas RA and RV wall damage was rare. Hospital mortality was 36% in the group of patients undergoing rescue intervention. Only 44% of patients survived in a good condition and were discharged home [8]. Bashir et al. reported cardiac or venous injuries in 3% of TLE patients, but mean implant duration time was much longer than in the previous study, i.e., 10.8 years. Overall, cardiac tamponade as a devastating injury was detected in 84.8% of cases but no one of the surgeons used pericardiocentesis as a therapeutic modality and urgent sternotomy was performed. Mortality rate in this report was 12.1% [10].

The organization of our TLE teamwork in compliance with maximum patient safety regulations may explain the absence of procedure-related deaths among 1500 patients in spite of the very long mean implant duration time and a relatively frequent need for rescue surgery. Mandatory continuous TEE monitoring during all TLE procedures and measurements of vital signs such as direct arterial blood pressure and capnography allowed us to recognize a serious complication very early, gaining time for proper rescue intervention. The excellent TLE organizational model solves the problem of complication-related deaths but has no or only a small influence on the development of major complications.

Damage to the tricuspid valve during extraction is estimated to range from 3.5% to 15%, and even to 19% [4,5,19–25]. In this study a clinically insignificant valve dysfunction was detected in 7.18% of cases, whereas significant TV damage that caused worsening TR by 2 or 3 degrees as compared to baseline (before TLE) occurred in 2.91% of patients, which is less than previously reported [4,5,19–25]. The need for surgical intervention in such cases is rare [19–25,31].

This study and available evidence [19–25,31] show that one of the most important TLE safety challenges is still the unsolved problem of TLE-related TV damage which is caused by fibrous adhesion of the lead to the TV leaflet. Excessive pulling on the lead may cause leaflet disruption, but also wrapping of the leaflet around the dilating sheath during rotational lead extraction. Excellent teamwork combined with TEE monitoring may help warn the extractor about potentially harmful situations leading to TV damage [27–30].

One should also bear in mind that the lead to be removed can be fused to the chordae tendineae or even to the head of the papillary muscle and damages to these structures may go unnoticed.

Continuous TEE monitoring during TLE facilitates the imaging of lead adhesion to the walls of the superior vena cava, tricuspid valve and walls of the right atrium and right ventricle, as well as assessing lead-to-lead adhesion [27]. In this aspect, real time transesophageal echocardiography for the guidance of transvenous lead extraction informs the operator about the danger of manipulations close to delicate cardiac structures and whether immediate modification to the plan of lead removal is necessary in order to prevent the occurrence of unwanted events [28,29]. In turn, postoperative TEE provides information about the results of TLE and helps establish further management [30].

5. Study Limitations

There are some limitations of this study. It is the experience of two high-volume centers and the same first operator. The database was prospectively integrated, but analysis was performed retrospectively. The TLE organizational model has not changed since 2015 and takes into account a comprehensive list of safety precautions (hybrid room, cardiac surgeon as co-operator, TEE monitoring, general anesthesia, arterial line etc.). All procedures were performed using all types of mechanical sheaths, but not laser powered sheaths. On the basis of our previous experience (2006–2014) we abstained from pericardiocentesis as a rule to avoid additional risk of complications and delay in open heart surgery as the most effective option.

6. Conclusions

Despite the long implant duration time (112.1 months) satisfying outcomes of lead extraction without procedure-related deaths (clinical success 98.93%, procedural success 96.13%) can be achieved using mechanical tools on condition that optimal safety precautions (immediate diagnosis of the event and rescue surgery) are taken into account. The absence of clinical and procedural success is caused by lead remnants or severe worsening of tricuspid regurgitation.

Major complications of TLE are unavoidable and may develop even in 2.20% of cases, minor complications are more frequent (7.67%). Major complications include cardiac laceration/vascular wall tear (1.40%) and severe tricuspid valve damage (0.80%).

The most frequent location of cardiac laceration/vascular wall tear is RAA(Right atrial appendage) (0.35%), connection of RA to VCS (0.33%) and VCS (0.20%). Other tear locations are rare. RAA, connection of RA to VCS and VCS are most frequent locations of CVWT requiring surgical repair (76.19% of cardiovascular wall injury).

Injury to structures other than RA (CS, SVC, connection of RA to IVC) was associated with higher drops in arterial blood pressure and CO^2 in exhaled air and much higher blood losses.

The most frequent minor complications were tricuspid valve damage (3.07%), pericardial effusion not requiring pericardiocentesis or surgical intervention (1.60%). Less frequent was blood transfusion related to blood loss during surgery, hematoma at the surgical site requiring drainage and pneumothorax.

Worsening of TR after TLE by one degree is a frequent finding (7.18%), worsening by 2 degrees (2.37%) and 3 degrees (0.542%) is rare, but the latter two may require surgery (leaflet repair with TV replacement) or strict follow-up.

The main TLE-related problem is still worsening TR (due to its long-term consequences) but not cardiac/vascular wall damage when non-powered mechanical sheaths are used as the first-line tools.

Author Contributions: Ł.T.—writing-original draft preparation; A.P.—investigation; W.J.—methodology, statistical study, D.N.—data curation, K.T.—data curation; P.S.—data curation; J.K.—investigation, K.D.—investigation, M.P.—data curation, A.K.—writing-review and editing. All authors have read and agreed to the published version of the manuscript.

Funding: This research received no external funding.

Institutional Review Board Statement: The study was conducted according to the guidelines of the Declaration of Helsinki, and approved by the of Bioethics Committee at the Regional Medical Chamber in Lublin protocol number 288/2018/KB/VII.

Informed Consent Statement: Informed consent was obtained from all subjects involved in the study.

Data Availability Statement: Readers can access the data supporting the conclusions of the study at www.usuwanieelektrod.pl (accessed on 11 September 2021).

Conflicts of Interest: Authors declare no conflict of interest.

References

1. Love, C.J.; Wilkoff, B.L.; Byrd, C.L.; Belott, P.H.; Brinker, J.A.; Fearnot, N.E.; Friedman, R.A.; Furman, S.; Goode, L.B.; Hayes, D.L.; et al. Recommendations for extraction of chronically implanted transvenous pacing and defibrillator leads: Indications, facilities, training. North American Society of Pacing and Electrophysiology Lead Extraction Conference Faculty. *Pacing Clin Electrophysiol.* **2000**, *23*, 544–551.
2. Wilkoff, B.L.; Love, C.J.; Byrd, C.L.; Bongiorni, M.G.; Carrillo, R.G.; Crossley, G.H.; Epstein, L.M.; Friedman, R.A.; Heart Rhythm Society; American Heart Association; et al. Transvenous lead extraction: Heart Rhythm Society expert consensus on facilities, training, indications, and patient management: This document was endorsed by the American Heart Association (AHA). *Heart Rhythm* **2009**, *6*, 1085–1104. [CrossRef] [PubMed]
3. Deharo, J.C.; Bongiorni, M.G.; Rozkovec, A.; Bracke, F.; Defaye, P.; Fernandez-Lozano, I.; Golzio, P.G.; Hansky, B.; Kennergren, C.; Manolis, A.S.; et al. Pathways for training and accreditation for transvenous lead extraction: A European Heart Rhythm Association position paper. *Europace* **2012**, *14*, 124–134.
4. Kusumoto, F.M.; Schoenfeld, M.H.; Wilkoff, B.; Berul, C.I.; Birgersdotter-Green, U.M.; Carrillo, R.; Cha, Y.M.; Clancy, J.; Deharo, J.C.; Ellenbogen, K.A.; et al. 2017 HRS expert consensus statement on cardiovascular implantable electronic device lead management and extraction. *Heart Rhythm* **2017**, *14*, e503–e551. [CrossRef]
5. Bongiorni, M.G.; Burri, H.; Deharo, J.C.; Starck, C.; Kennergren, C.; Saghy, L.; Rao, A.; Tascini, C.; Lever, N.; Kutarski, A.; et al. 2018 EHRA expert consensus statement on lead extraction: Recommendations on definitions, endpoints, research trial design, and data collection requirements for clinical scientific studies and registries: Endorsed by APHRS/HRS/LAHRS. *Europace* **2018**, *20*, 1217. [CrossRef] [PubMed]
6. Kołodzińska, A.; Kutarski, A.; Koperski, Ł.; Grabowski, M.; Małecka, B.; Opolski, G. Differences in encapsulating lead tissue in patients who underwent transvenous lead removal. *Europace* **2012**, *14*, 994–1001. [CrossRef]
7. Nowosielecka, D.; Polewczyk, A.; Jacheć, W.; Tułecki, Ł.; Kleinrok, A.; Kutarski, A. Echocardiographic findings in patients with cardiac implantable electronic devices-analysis of factors predisposing to lead-associated changes. *Clin. Physiol. Funct. Imaging* **2021**, *41*, 25–41. [CrossRef] [PubMed]
8. Brunner, M.P.; Cronin, E.M.; Wazni, O.; Baranowski, B.; Saliba, W.I.; Sabik, J.F.; Lindsay, B.D.; Wilkoff, B.L.; Tarakji, K.G. Outcomes of patients requiring emergent surgical or endovascular intervention for catastrophic complications during transvenous lead extraction. *Heart Rhythm* **2014**, *11*, 419–425. [CrossRef] [PubMed]
9. Wang, W.; Wang, X.; Modry, D.; Wang, S. Cardiopulmonary bypass standby avoids fatality due to vascular laceration in laser-assisted lead extraction. *J. Card. Surg.* **2014**, *29*, 274–278. [CrossRef]
10. Bashir, J.; Fedoruk, L.M.; Ofiesh, J.; Karim, S.S.; Tyers, G.F.O. Classification and Surgical Repair of Injuries Sustained During Transvenous Lead Extraction'. *Circ. Arrhythm. Electrophysiol.* **2016**, *9*, e003741.
11. Maus, T.M.; Shurter, J.; Nguyen, L.; Birgersdotter-Green, U.; Pretorius, V. Multidisciplinary approach to transvenous lead extraction: A single center's experience. *J. Cardiothorac. Vasc. Anesth.* **2015**, *29*, 265–270. [CrossRef]
12. Caniglia-Miller, J.M.; Bussey, W.D.; Kamtz, N.M.; Tsai, S.F.; Erickson, C.C.; Anderson, D.R.; Moulton, M.J. Surgical management of major intrathoracic hemorrhage resulting from high-risk transvenous pacemaker/defibrillator lead extraction. *J. Card Surg.* **2015**, *30*, 149–153. [CrossRef]
13. Hosseini, S.M.; Rozen, G.; Kaadan, M.I.; Galvin, J.; Ruskin, J.N. Safety and In-Hospital Outcomes of Transvenous Lead Extraction for Cardiac Implantable Device-Related Infections: Analysis of 13 Years of Inpatient Data in the United States. *JACC Clin. Electrophysiol.* **2019**, *5*, 1450–1458. [CrossRef] [PubMed]
14. Hauser, R.G.; Katsiyiannis, W.T.; Gornick, C.C.; Almquist, A.K.; Kallinen, L.M. Deaths and cardiovascular injuries due to device-assisted implantable cardioverter–defibrillator and pacemaker lead extraction. *Europace* **2010**, *1*, 395–401. [CrossRef]
15. Kutarski, A.; Czajkowski, M.; Pietura, R.; Obszanski, B.; Polewczyk, A.; Jachec, W.; Polewczyk, M.; Mlynarczyk, K.; Grabowski, M.; Opolski, G. Effectiveness, safety, and long-term outcomes of non-powered mechanical sheaths for transvenous lead extraction. *Europace* **2018**, *20*, 1324–1333. [CrossRef]
16. Issa, Z.F. Transvenous lead extraction in 1000 patients guided by intraprocedural risk stratification without surgical backup. *Heart Rhythm* **2021**, *18*, 1272–1278, online ahead of print. [CrossRef] [PubMed]

17. Roberto, M.; Sicuso, R.; Manganiello, S.; Catto, V.; Salvi, L.; Nafi, M.; Casella, M.; Rossi, F.; Grillo, F.; Saccocci, M.; et al. Cardiac surgeon and electrophysiologist shoulder-to-shoulder approach: Hybrid room, a kingdom for two. A zero mortality transvenous lead extraction single center experience. *Int. J. Cardiol.* **2019**, *279*, 35–39. [CrossRef] [PubMed]
18. Gaca, J.G.; Lima, B.; Milano, C.A.; Lin, S.S.; Davis, R.D.; Lowe, J.E.; Smith, P.K. Laser-assisted extraction of pacemaker and defibrillator leads: The role of the cardiac surgeon. *Ann. Thorac. Surg.* **2009**, *87*, 1446–1450. [CrossRef]
19. Park, S.J.; Gentry, J.L., 3rd; Varma, N.; Wazni, O.; Tarakji, K.G.; Mehta, A.; Mick, S.; Grimm, R.; Wilkoff, B.L. Transvenous Extraction of Pacemaker and Defibrillator Leads and the Risk of Tricuspid Valve Regurgitation. *JACC Clin. Electrophysiol.* **2018**, *4*, 1421–1428. [CrossRef] [PubMed]
20. Pecha, S.; Castro, L.; Gosau, N.; Linder, M.; Vogler, J.; Willems, S.; Reichenspurner, H.; Hakmi, S. Evaluation of tricuspid valve regurgitation following laser lead extraction. *Eur. J. Cardiothorac. Surg.* **2017**, *51*, 1108–1111. [CrossRef]
21. Givon, A.; Vedernikova, N.; Luria, D.; Vatury, O.; Kuperstein, R.; Feinberg, M.S.; Eldar, M.; Glikson, M.; Nof, E. Tricuspid Regurgitation following Lead Extraction: Risk Factors and Clinical Course. *Isr. Med. Assoc. J.* **2016**, *18*, 18–22.
22. Regoli, F.; Caputo, M.; Conte, G.; Faletra, F.F.; Moccetti, T.; Pasotti, E.; Cassina, T.; Casso, G.; Schlotterbeck, H.; Engeler, A.; et al. Clinical utility of routine use of continuous transesophageal echocardiography monitoring during transvenous lead extraction procedure. *Heart Rhythm* **2015**, *12*, 313–320. [CrossRef]
23. Coffey, J.O.; Sager, S.J.; Gangireddy, S.; Levine, A.; Viles-Gonzalez, J.F.; Fischer, A. The impact of transvenous lead extraction on tricuspid valve function. *Pacing Clin. Electrophysiol.* **2014**, *37*, 19–24. [CrossRef] [PubMed]
24. Rodriguez, Y.; Mesa, J.; Arguelles, E.; Carrillo, R.G. Tricuspid insufficiency after laser lead extraction. *Pacing Clin. Electrophysiol.* **2013**, *36*, 939–944. [CrossRef]
25. Franceschi, F.; Thuny, F.; Giorgi, R.; Sanaa, I.; Peyrouse, E.; Assouan, X.; Prévôt, S.; Bastard, E.; Habib, G.; Deharo, J.C. Incidence, risk factors, and outcome of traumatic tricuspid regurgitation after percutaneous ventricular lead removal. *J. Am. Coll. Cardiol.* **2009**, *53*, 2168–2174. [CrossRef]
26. Jacheć, W.; Polewczyk, A.; Polewczyk, M.; Tomasik, A.; Kutarski, A. Transvenous Lead Extraction SAFeTY Score for Risk Stratification and Proper Patient Selection for Removal Procedures Using Mechanical Tools. *J. Clin. Med.* **2020**, *9*, 361. [CrossRef] [PubMed]
27. Nowosielecka, D.; Jacheć, W.; Polewczyk, A.; Tułecki, Ł.; Tomków, K.; Stefańczyk, P.; Tomaszewski, A.; Brzozowski, W.; Szcześniak-Stańczyk, D.; Kleinrok, A.; et al. Transesophageal Echocardiography as a Monitoring Tool during Transvenous Lead Extraction-does It Improve Procedure Effectiveness? *J. Clin. Med.* **2020**, *9*, 1382. [CrossRef]
28. Nowosielecka, D.; Polewczyk, A.; Jacheć, W.; Tułecki, Ł.; Tomków, K.; Stefańczyk, P.; Kleinrok, A.; Kutarski, A. A new approach to the continuous monitoring of transvenous lead extraction using transesophageal echocardiography-Analysis of 936 procedures. *Echocardiography* **2020**, *37*, 601–611. [CrossRef]
29. Nowosielecka, D.; Polewczyk, A.; Jacheć, W.; Kleinrok, A.; Tułecki, Ł.; Kutarski, A. Transesophageal echocardiography for the monitoring of transvenous lead extraction. *Kardiol. Pol.* **2020**, *78*, 1206–1214. [CrossRef] [PubMed]
30. Nowosielecka, D.; Jacheć, W.; Polewczyk, A.; Kleinrok, A.; Tułecki, Ł.; Kutarski, A. The prognostic value of transesophageal echocardiography after transvenous lead extraction: Landscape after battle. *Cardiovasc. Diagn. Ther.* **2021**, *11*, 394–410. [CrossRef]
31. Mehrotra, D.; Kejriwal, N.K. Tricuspid valve repair for torrential tricuspid regurgitation after permanent pacemaker lead extraction. *Tex. Heart Inst. J.* **2011**, *38*, 305–307. [PubMed]

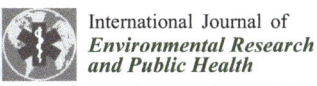

Article

The Influence of Lead-Related Venous Obstruction on the Complexity and Outcomes of Transvenous Lead Extraction

Marek Czajkowski [1], Wojciech Jacheć [2], Anna Polewczyk [3,4,*], Jarosław Kosior [5], Dorota Nowosielecka [6], Łukasz Tułecki [7], Paweł Stefańczyk [6] and Andrzej Kutarski [8]

1. Department of Cardiac Surgery, Medical University of Lublin Poland, 20-078 Lublin, Poland; mczajkowski@interia.pl
2. 2nd Department of Cardiology, Faculty of Medical Science in Zabrze, Medical University of Silesia, Zabrze, 40-055 Katowice, Poland; wjachec@interia.pl
3. Department of Physiology, Pathophysiology and Clinical Immunology, Collegium Medicum of Jan Kochanowski University, 25-736 Kielce, Poland
4. Department of Cardiac Surgery, Świętokrzyskie Cardiology Center, 25-736 Kielce, Poland
5. Department of Cardiology, Masovian Specialistic Hospital, 26-617 Radom, Poland; jaroslaw.kosior@icloud.com
6. Department of Cardiology, The Pope John Paul II Province Hospital, 22-400 Zamość, Poland; dornowos@wp.pl (D.N.); paolost@interia.pl (P.S.)
7. Department of Cardiac Surgery, The Pope John Paul II Province Hospital, 22-400 Zamość, Poland; luke27@poczta.onet.pl
8. Department of Cardiology, Medical University of Lublin Poland, 20-078 Lublin, Poland; a_kutarski@yahoo.com
* Correspondence: annapolewczyk@wp.pl; Tel.: +48-6-0002-4074

Abstract: Background: Little is known about lead-related venous stenosis/occlusion (LRVSO), and the influence of LRVSO on the complexity and outcomes of transvenous lead extraction (TLE) is debated in the literature. Methods: We performed a retrospective analysis of venograms from 2909 patients who underwent TLE between 2008 and 2021 at a high-volume center. Results: Advanced LRVSO was more common in elderly men with a high Charlson comorbidity index. Procedure duration, extraction of superfluous leads, occurrence of any technical difficulty, lead-to-lead binding, fracture of the lead being extracted, need to use alternative approach and lasso catheters or metal sheaths were found to be associated with LRVSO. The presence of LRVSO had no impact on the number of major complications including TLE-related tricuspid valve damage. The achievement of complete procedural or clinical success did not depend on the presence of LRVSO. Long-term mortality, in contrast to periprocedural and short-term mortality, was significantly worse in the groups with LRSVO. Conclusions: LRVSO can be considered as an additional TLE-related risk factor. The effect of LRVSO on major complications including periprocedural mortality and on short-term mortality has not been established. However, LRVSO has been associated with poor long-term survival.

Keywords: lead-related venous obstruction; transvenous lead extraction; lead extraction complications; lead extraction complexity

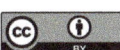

1. Background

Permanent cardiac pacing remains the leading treatment for patients with various rhythm disorders, conduction disturbances and ventricular arrhythmias. In recent years, we have also observed an increase in the implantation of more complex devices used in the prevention of sudden cardiac death and in the treatment of severe heart failure. In spite of technological progress over the last decade, conventional pacemakers, implantable cardioverter-defibrillators and cardiac resynchronization therapy (PM/ICD/CRT) devices still have endocardial leads. However, after the beginning of the endocardial pacing era only a few studies have investigated lead-related venous stenosis/occlusion (LRVSO) [1–20]. Various lead-related problems (infectious and non-infectious) are an inherent component of permanent endocardial pacing, and transvenous lead extraction (TLE) is considered an essential technique in lead management strategy [21–24]. TLE is a complex procedure that sometimes may lead to fatal complications such as venous or cardiac injury. Carrying out the procedure is often associated with technical problems and requires additional approaches and tools [22–25]. There are numerous reports on the estimation of the real risk of the TLE [26–29] but none of them considered LRVSO as a predictor of procedure difficulties. Among twenty reports on LRVSO [1–20], only three papers analyzed the occurrence of LRVSO before TLE [2,6,14], and only two considered the influence of LRVSO on procedure complexity providing at the same time conflicting results. Among 20 reports on LRVSO only two studies were carried out in populations over 200 patients [1,2], 10 in 100–150 participants [3–12] and the remaining eight studies in populations consisting of 30–89 patients [13–20]. In this study, a total of 2909 TLE procedures were preceded by venography and LRVSO was documented in 2138 venograms. Ipsilateral venography before TLE is an integral part of the procedure (in the absence of contraindications for contrast intake).

Goal of the Study

The aim of this study was to determine the incidence of varying degrees of LRVSO and to examine the influence of LRVSO on procedure difficulty, complexity, major complications related to TLE, procedure effectiveness as well as mid- and long-term mortality after TLE.

2. Methods

2.1. Study Population

A post-hoc analysis of clinical data from 2909 patients undergoing transvenous lead extraction (TLE) between June 2008 and March 2021 at a single high-volume center was performed. All information regarding the patients and the procedures were entered into the computer database on a current basis. Patients with medical contraindications for venography (contrast intake) were excluded from the study.

Table 1 summarizes the most important information regarding the study population.

Table 1. Characteristics of the study group.

All Patients (2909)	Mean/Number	SD/%
Patient age during TLE [years]	66.90	13.99
Patient age at first implantation [years]	58.51	15.67
Sex (% of female patients)	1147	39.43%
Etiology: IHD, MI	1676	57.61%
Etiology: cardiomyopathy, valvular heart disease	448	15.40%
Etiology: congenital, channelopathies, neurocardiogenic, post cardiac surgery	784	26.95%
LVEF [%]	48.89	15.21
Renal failure (any)	607	20.87%
Previous sternotomy	435	14.95%
Charlson comorbidity index [number of points]	4.775	3.625
Systemic infection (with pocket infection or not)	599	20.59%
Local (pocket) infection	253	8.70%
Lead failure (replacement)	1505	57.74%

Table 1. Cont.

All Patients (2909)	Mean/Number	SD/%
Change of pacing mode/upgrading, downgrading	176	6.05%
Other (abandoned lead/prevention of abandonment (AF, superfluous leads), threatening/potentially threatening lead (loops, free ending, left heart, LDTD), other (MRI indications, cancer, painful pocket, loss of indications for pacing/ICD), regaining venous access (symptomatic occlusion, SVC syndrome, lead replacement/upgrading)	374	12.86%
System: pacemaker (any)	2013	69.20%
System: ICD-V, ICD-D	281	22.93%
System: CRT-D	667	7.80%
Dwell time of the oldest lead per patient before TLE [months]	101.5	75.57
Cumulative lead dwell time before TLE [years]	15.31	12.925
Major complications: all	61	2.10%
Major complications (with rescue cardiac surgery)	35	1.20%
Major complications (without rescue cardiac surgery)	7	1.20%
Minor complications	174	5.98%

AF—atrial fibrillation, CRT-D: implantable cardioverter-defibrillator with resynchronization function, ICD—implantable cardioverter-defibrillator, ICD-D—dual chamber implantable cardioverter-defibrillator, ICD-V—single chamber implantable cardioverter-defibrillator, IHD—ischemic heart disease, LDTD—lead-dependent tricuspid dysfunction, LVEF—left ventricular ejection fraction, MI—myocardial infarction, MRI—magnetic resonance imaging, SVC—superior vena cava, TLE—transvenous lead extraction.

The current study uses data from a high-volume center that performs more than 200 TLE per year.

The percentage of serious complications is relatively higher compared to other reports, however, in the presented center, the most difficult procedures in the country are performed.

The first line tools used in study center are conventional mechanical sheaths, powered rotational mechanical sheaths and other instruments are second-line tools. Excimer laser sheaths are not used.

2.2. Venography

Preoperative venography was performed in 2909 patients submitted for transvenous lead extraction between June 2008 and March 2021 at our high-volume center. A peripheral intravenous catheter was placed in the peripheral arm vein on the side (or both sides of the chest) to be examined. All patients received an injection of 20–40 mL high-quality contrast medium (350 mg iodine/mL) Iomeron 350 into the peripheral arm vein on the side of endocardial lead implantation. Venous blood flow in the upper arm, neck and chest was recorded by cine-angiography. All images were acquired in the anteroposterior view. The venograms were obtained in a single plane (anterior–posterior) and stored on CD-ROM discs. An experienced cardiologist and experienced (trained by an interventional radiologist) cardiac surgeon reviewed the venograms, and venous patency was graded on a five-degree scale from normal flow to complete occlusion. All venograms were obtained in the same manner. Venographic analysis: at baseline, the narrowest and widest points of the target vessel for lead placement were identified by visual inspection to obtain minimum and maximum venous diameters, and measurements from two to three individually calibrated frames were averaged to determine the final status of the vein as no stenosis, mild stenosis (<50% narrowing), moderate stenosis (50–80% narrowing), severe stenosis ($\geq$80% narrowing) and complete occlusion of the axillary (AxV), subclavian (ScV), innominate (brachiocephalic) (AnV) veins and superior vena cava (SVC). In spite of contrast injection in the arm vein on the side of the endocardial lead, regional collateral blood vessels and venous collateral blood flow in the neck enabled evaluation of the brachiocephalic vein on the opposite side of the chest. What is the significance of this classification of vessel narrowing in clinical practice? LVRSO was graded according to our own, arbitrarily estimated, criteria, which rely to the remaining effective vein lumen necessary for different electrodes/catheters safe passage.

Mild narrowing: possible insertion of a new/additional lead using standard introducers, central venous catheters, permanent catheters for hemodialysis and there is a chance that the arteriovenous (AV) fistula will work properly.

Moderate narrowing: probable insertion of a new lead but hydrophilic guide wires and longer introducers are necessary, possible insertion of central venous catheters (troubles possible), possible insertion of permanent catheters for hemodialysis and there is a small chance that the AV fistula will work properly.

Severe narrowing: impossible insertion of a new lead, hydrophilic guide wires and longer introducers might be helpful, insertion of central venous catheters may be risky, chances to pass a catheter for hemodialysis without venoplasty are very small and there is no chance that the AV fistula will work properly.

Complete occlusion: no chance to pass a hydrophilic guide wire; only lead extraction and regaining venous access enables the insertion of a new lead.

Reuse of occluded veins and technical aspects of lead extraction/replacement depend not only on maximal venous narrowing but also on the length of the narrowing (the number of the affected vessels, too).

2.3. Lead Extraction Procedure

Lead extraction procedures were defined according to the most recent guidelines on management of lead-related complications (HRS 2017 and EHRA 2018) [21–23]. Indications for TLE and type of periprocedural complications were defined according to the 2017 HRS Expert Consensus Statement on Cardiovascular Implantable Electronic Device Lead Management and Extraction [22].

All procedures were performed using non-powered mechanical systems such as polypropylene Byrd dilator sheaths (Cook® Medical, Leechburg, PA, USA), mainly via the implant vein. If technical difficulties arose, alternative venous approaches and/or additional tools such as Evolution (Cook® Medical, Leechburg, PA, USA), TightRail (Spectranetix, Colorado Springs, CO, USA), lassos, basket catheters were used. Excimer laser sheaths were not used.

All extraction procedures were performed following different organizational models spanning 25 years of experience. In the initial era of lead extraction, the procedures were performed in the electrophysiology laboratory using intravenous analgesia/sedation; then the recommended safety precautions were observed to perform more complex and risky procedures in the operating theater, and finally in the hybrid room under general anesthesia. The core extraction team has consisted of the same very experienced TLE operator and a dedicated cardiac surgeon with an experienced echocardiographist over the last six years.

2.4. TEE Monitoring during TLE

TTE, pre- and postoperative TEE were mandatory (excluding contraindications) from the very beginning. Continuous transesophageal echocardiographic (TEE) monitoring has been an important standard tool over the last six years [30–32]. TEE in our series was performed using Philips iE33 or GE Vivid S 70 machines equipped with X7-2t Live 3D or 6VT-D probes. All recordings were archived and consisted of pre-procedural examination, navigation of lead removal and post-procedural evaluation of the efficacy of the procedure with an assessment of possible complications [30–32]. The intra-procedural phase of TEE monitoring allowed visualization of pulling on the cardiac walls and invagination of the right ventricle during lead removal, followed by a drop in systolic blood pressure in response to this maneuver. Continuous monitoring made it possible to clarify the cause of blood pressure fall during TLE [30–32].

2.5. Statistical Analysis

The Shapiro–Wilk test showed that most continuous variables were normally distributed. For uniformity, all continuous variables are presented as the mean ± standard deviation. The categorical variables are presented as number and percentage. In the first step the Kruskal–Wallis ANOVA test was used to determine whether there were statistically significant differences between groups. Next, the variables achieving $p < 0.1$ were compared using the nonparametric Chi^2 test with Yates correction (dichotomous data) or the unpaired Mann–Whitney U test (continuous data), as appropriate. Comparisons were made between Groups 1 and 2 vs. Groups 4 and 5. A p-value less than 0.05 was considered as statistically significant. In order to assess the effect of LRVSO on mortality, Kaplan–Meier survival curves were plotted, the course of which was assessed using the log rank test. Statistical analysis was performed with Statistica version 13.3 (TIBCO Software Inc., Palo Alto, CA, USA).

2.6. Approval of the Bioethics Committee

All patients gave their informed written consent to undergo TLE and use anonymous data from their medical records, approved by the Bioethics Committee at the Regional Chamber of Physicians in Lublin No. 288/2018/KB/VII. The study was carried out in accordance with the ethical standards of the 1964 Declaration of Helsinki.

3. Results

Patient Groups

For the purposes of analysis, the study population was divided into five groups according to venogram results, namely Group 1—no stenosis (499 patients), 2—mild stenosis (574 pts), 3—moderate stenosis (605 pts), 4—severe stenosis (581 pts) and 5—total occlusion (650 pts). Only maximal venous narrowing was considered as a criterion in patient selection.

Tables 2–4 summarize specific patient-, system- and procedure-related risk factors for procedure complexity, efficacy, complications and long-term mortality after TLE.

Analysis of the clinical factors demonstrated that lead-related stenosis/occlusion correlated with patient age during TLE, male gender and Charlson comorbidity index. Other patient-related risk factors for major complications, i.e., indications for CIED implantation, functional NYHA class III and IV, decreased LVEF, renal failure and previous sternotomy were not related to LRVSO (Table 2).

Analysis of CIED systems and history of pacing showed that venous stenosis or lead-related (LR) total venous occlusion were more frequent in CRT-D recipients. Patients with ICD (VVI, DDD) were less likely, albeit insignificantly to have total venous occlusion.

Patients with redundant loops of the lead before TLE, leads with proximal end in the coronary sinus vein (CSV) and a higher number of CIED-related procedures before lead extraction were more likely to have severe venous stenosis or total occlusion.

Patients with severe venous stenosis or LR total venous occlusion had more risk factors for major complications (MC) and higher procedure complexity estimated with the SAFeTY TLE calculator [26]. These patients also had multiple leads to be removed (including three or more leads), they were more likely to require venous approach on both sides of the chest, extraction of leads with redundant loops in the heart, extraction of abandoned lead (s) and extraction of lead (s) with long or very long implant duration (Table 2).

Table 2. Patient-, system- and procedure-related risk factors for procedure complexity and major complications.

	No Stenosis 1	Mild Stenosis 2	Moderate Stenosis 3	Severe Stenosis 4	Total Occlusion 5	ANOVA Kruskal–Wallis Test (1–5) p	Mann–Whitney U/Chi² Tests (1–2) vs. (4–5)
Number of Patients	N = 499 (17.15%)	N = 574 (19.73%)	N = 605 (20.80%)	N = 581 (19.97%)	N = 650 (22.34%)		
	Mean ± SD n (%)	Mean ± SD n (%)	Mean ± SD n (%)	Mean ± SD n (%)	Mean ± SD n (%)		
Patient-related risk factors for TLE complexity and complications							
Patient age during TLE [years]	64.48 ± 14.85	66.74 ± 13.69	66.64 ± 13.79	68.57 ± 13.04	67.68 ± 14.32	<0.001	<0.001
Male gender	325 (65.13)	324 (56.44)	324 (53.55)	342 (58.86)	447 (68.77)	<0.001	0.019
Etiology: IHD, MI	278 (55.71)	329 (57.31)	353 (58.34)	361 (62.13)	355 (54.62)	0.112	
Etiology: non-ischemic	221 (44.29)	245 (42.69)	252 (41.66)	220 (37.87)	295 (45.38)	0.112	
NYHA class III and IV (%)	67 (13.42)	96 (16.72)	71 (11.73)	196 (33.74)	99 (15.23)	0.523	
LVEF < 40%	158 (31.66)	173 (30.14)	177 (29.26)	196 (33.74)	215 (33.08)	0.847	
Renal failure (any)	88 (17.64)	119 (20.73)	122 (20.17)	121 (20.83)	156 (24.00)	0.211	
Previous sternotomy	81 (16.23)	85 (14.81)	79 (13.06)	76 (13.08)	114 (17.54)	0.210	
Charlson comorbidity index [number of points]	4.543 ± 3.789	4.702 ± 3.380	4.688 ± 3.589	5.086 ± 3.629	4.728 ± 3.550	0.038	0.016
CIED system and history of pacing							
Device type—pacemaker (any)	350 (70.14)	402 (70.04)	416 (68.76)	384 (66.09)	461 (70.92)	0.193	
Device type—ICD-V, ICD-D	126 (25.25)	127 (22.13)	144 (23.80)	141 (24.27)	127 (19.54)	0.142	
Device type—CRT-D	21 (4.208)	44 (7.666)	44 (7.237)	56 (9.639)	62 (9.54)	0.006	0.002
Redundant loop of the lead on X-Rays before TLE	20 (4.01)	21 (3.659)	25 (4.132)	26 (4.475)	44 (6.769)	0.074	0.047
Lead with proximal end in CVS before TLE	9 (1.804)	10 (1.742)	7 (1.150)	11 (1.893)	14 (2.154)	<0.001	0.762
Number of CIED-related procedures before TLE (SD)	1.728 ± 0.970	1.701 ± 0.881	1.777 ± 1.068	1.806 ± 0.959	2.088 ± 1.300	<0.001	<0.001
TLE before current TLE	23 (4.609)	23 (4.007)	19 (3.140)	27 (4.647)	39 (6.00)	0.200	
Risk factors for major complications and procedure complexity							

Table 2. Cont.

	No Stenosis 1	Mild Stenosis 2	Moderate Stenosis 3	Severe Stenosis 4	Total Occlusion 5	ANOVA Kruskal–Wallis Test (1–5) p	Mann–Whitney U/Chi^2 Tests (1–2) vs. (4–5)
Number of Patients	N = 499 (17.15%)	N = 574 (19.73%)	N = 605 (20.80%)	N = 581 (19.97%)	N = 650 (22.34%)		
	Mean ± SD n (%)	Mean ± SD n (%)	Mean ± SD n (%)	Mean ± SD n (%)	Mean ± SD n (%)		
Number of extracted leads per patient [n]	1.597 ± 0.619	1.582 ± 0.681	1.623 ± 0.666	1.683 ± 0.719	1.835 ± 0.880	<0.001	<0.001
Three or more leads extracted	30 (6.012)	46 (8.014)	55 (9.090)	73 (12.57)	113 (17.38)	<0.001	<0.001
Approach: left	483 (96.79)	551 (95.99)	578 (95.54)	548 (94.32)	599 (92.15)	0.002	<0.001
Approach: right	7 (1.403)	9 (1.568)	12 (1.980)	17 (2.930)	11 (1.690)	0.443	
Approach: both	1 (0.200)	3 (0.523)	3 (0.496)	5 (0.860)	14 (2.154)	0.003	0.009
Approach: femoral	1 (0.200)	2 (0.348)	2 (0.331)	0 (0.00)	6 (0.923)	0.225	
Approach: subclavian-femoral	3 (0.601)	4 (0.697)	3 (0.496)	2 (0.344)	5 (0.970)	0.581	
Approach: other, combined	4 (0.802)	3 (0.523)	5 (0.826)	9 (1.549)	14 (2.150)	0.061	0.017
Approach: Jugular	0 (0.00)	2 (0.348)	0 (0.00)	0 (0.00)	0 (0.00)	0.086	0.420
Extraction of leads with redundant loop	14 (2.806)	14 (2.439)	20 (3.306)	21 (3.614)	37 (5.690)	0.026	0.011
Extraction of broken lead with proximal end in CS	11 (2.204)	11 (1.916)	7 (1.157)	10 (1.721)	16 (2.460)	0.756	
Extraction of abandoned lead(s) (any)	35 (7.014)	45 (7.840)	39 (6.446)	60 (10.33)	102 (15.69)	<0.001	<0.001
Extraction of abandoned lead(s) [n]	0.074 ± 0.277	0.103 ± 0.380	0.083 ± 0.340	0.138 ± 0.441	0.208 ± 0.520	<0.001	<0.001
Oldest extracted lead (months)	96.25 ± 73.71	102.4 ± 74.46	100.3 ± 76.37	94.21 ± 70.22	104.86 ± 76.70	0.078	
Average (per patient) extracted lead dwell time [months]	92.24 ± 67.47	97.85 ± 67.97	95.38 ± 70.31	88.59 ± 62.52	96.49 ± 67.68	0.163	
Cumulative dwell time of extracted leads [years]	12.30 ± 12.11	13.57 ± 12.43	13.55 ± 12.47	12.98 ± 11.59	15.39 ± 14.13	0 < 0.001	0.008
SAFeTY TLE calculator of risk for MC [points]	5.290 ± 4.117	5.828 ± 4.130	5.995 ± 4.249	5.597 ± 4.090	6.333 ± 4.560	0.002	<0.024
SAFeTY TLE calculator of risk for MC [%]	1.470 ± 2.566	1.621 ± 2.490	1.782 ± 3.430	1.608 ± 2.690	2.089 ± 3.650	0.002	<0.001

CRTD—implantable cardioverter-defibrillator with resynchronization function, CS—coronary sinus, ICD-D—dual chamber implantable cardioverter-defibrillator, ICD-V—single chamber implantable cardioverter-defibrillator, IHD—ischemic heart disease, LVEF—left ventricular ejection fraction, MI—myocardial infarction, NYHA—New York Heart Association functional class, TLE—transvenous lead extraction.

Table 3. TLE complexity.

	No Stenosis 1	Mild Stenosis 2	Moderate Stenosis 3	Severe Stenosis 4	Total Occlusion 5	ANOVA Kruskal–Wallis Test (1–5) p	ANOVA Kruskal–Wallis Test (1–2) vs. (4–5)
Number of Patients	N = 499	N = 574	N = 605	N = 581	N = 650		
	Mean ± SD n (%)	Mean ± SD n (%)	Mean ± SD n (%)	Mean ± SD n (%)	Mean ± SD n (%)		
TLE complexity							
Procedure duration (skin-to-skin) [minutes]	57.66 ± 22.54	59.18 ± 25.99	58.23 ± 20.90	59.33 ± 24.09	64.16 ± 33.85	0.018	0.075
Procedure duration (sheath-to-sheath) [minutes]	12.36 ± 19.06	13.26 ± 21.86	12.73 ± 17.14	13.56 ± 20.36	20.32 ± 32.45	<0.001	<0.001
Average time of single lead extraction [minutes]	8.149 ± 11.26	8.441 ± 15.05	7.755 ± 9.616	7.568 ± 8.884	10.56 ± 15.30	<0.001	0.126
All leads were extracted	399 (79.96)	432 (75.26)	450 (74.38)	420 (72.29)	503 (77.38)	0.040	0.181
Functional lead was left in place for continuous use	98 (19.64)	137 (23.87)	153 (25.29)	157 (27.02)	141 (21.69)	0.030	0.207
Non-functional lead was left in place	1 (0.200)	3 (0.523)	1 (0.165)	1 (0.172)	6 (0.923)	0.302	
Non-functional superfluous lead was extracted	35 (7.014)	45 (7.840)	39 (6.446)	60 (10.33)	102 (15.69)	<0.001	<0.001
Technical problem during TLE (any)	85 (17.03)	110 (19.16)	116 (19.17)	109 (18.76)	162 (24.92)	0.011	0.025
Block in implant vein (subclavian region)	34 (6.814)	39 (6.794)	48 (7.934)	43 (7.401)	65 (10.00)	0.154	
Lead-to-lead binding	28 (5.611)	33 (5.749)	39 (6.446)	42 (7.229)	64 (9.846)	0.030	0.009
Byrd dilator collapse/torsion/"fracture"	16 (3.206)	19 (3.310)	19 (3.140)	19 (3.270)	23 (3.538)	0.968	
Lead fracture during extraction	22 (4.409)	22 (3.833)	31 (5.124)	29 (4.991)	51 (7.846)	0.004	0.014
Need to change venous approach	12 (2.405)	13 (2.265)	14 (2.314)	18 (3.098)	41 (6.308)	<0.001	<0.002
Functional lead dislodgement	6 (1.202)	8 (1.394)	6 (0.992)	5 (0.861)	5 (0.769)	0.824	

Table 3. Cont.

	No Stenosis 1	Mild Stenosis 2	Moderate Stenosis 3	Severe Stenosis 4	Total Occlusion 5	ANOVA Kruskal–Wallis Test (1–5) p	ANOVA Kruskal–Wallis Test (1–2) vs. (4–5)
Number of Patients	N = 499	N = 574	N = 605	N = 581	N = 650		
	Mean ± SD n (%)	Mean ± SD n (%)	Mean ± SD n (%)	Mean ± SD n (%)	Mean ± SD n (%)		
Loss of lead fragment	2 (0.401)	8 (1.394)	6 (0.992)	5 (0.861)	5 (0.769)	0.800	
Reel of ICD lead coil	2 (0.401)	4 (0.697)	5 (0.826)	1 (0.172)	2 (0.308)	0.222	
Number of big technical problems	1.316 ± 0.637	1.325 ± 0.718	1.313 ± 0.685	1.330 ± 0.620	1.500 ± 0.784	0.002	0.053
One technical problem only	57 (11.42)	65 (11.32)	76 (12.56)	64 (11.01)	81 (12.46)	0.925	
Two technical problems	16 (3.206)	12 (2.091)	12 (1.983)	21 (3.614)	33 (5.077)	0.006	0.029
Three or more technical problems	3 (0.601)	6 (1.045)	8 (1.322)	3 (0.515)	14 (2.154)	<0.001	0.302
Other smaller technical problems	25 (5.010)	23 (4.007)	26 (4.298)	22 (3.787)	49 (7.538)	0.003	0.192
Use of additional tools							
Evolution (old and new) or tight rail	7 (1.403)	5 (0.871)	8 (1.322)	7 (1.205)	17 (2.615)	0.121	
Metal sheath	30 (6.012)	36 (6.272)	50 (8.264)	40 (6.886)	63 (9.692)	0.064	0.051
Lasso catheter/snare	14 (2.806)	13 (2.265)	17 (2.810)	17 (2.926)	33 (5.077)	0.017	0.052
Basket catheter	7 (1.403)	6 (1.045)	4 (0.661)	2 (0.344)	8 (1.231)	0.284	

ICD—implantable cardioverter-defibrillator, TLE—transvenous lead extraction.

Table 4. TLE efficacy and complications, and long-term mortality after TLE.

	No Stenosis 1	Mild Stenosis 2	Moderate Stenosis 3	Severe Stenosis 4	Total Occlusion 5	ANOVA Kruskal–Wallis Test (1–5) p	ANOVA Kruskal–Wallis Test (1–2) vs. (4–5)
Number of Patients	N = 499	N = 574	N = 605	N = 581	N = 650		
	Mean ± SD n (%)	Mean ± SD n (%)	Mean ± SD n (%)	Mean ± SD n (%)	Mean ± SD n (%)		
TLE efficacy and complications							
Major complications (any)	8 (1.603)	10 (1.742)	11 (1.818)	16 (2.754)	16 (2.461)	0.599	
Hemopericardium	5 (1.002)	6 (1.045)	8 (1.322)	11 (1.893)	9 (1.385)	0.707	
Hemothorax	3 (0.601)	3 (0.523)	1 (0.165)	0 (0.00)	3 (0.462)	0.288	
Tricuspid valve damage during TLE	2 (0.401)	4 (0.697)	2 (0.331)	5 (0.861)	3 (0.462)	0.722	
Rescue cardiac surgery	4 (0.802)	3 (0.523)	8 (1.322)	9 (1.549)	10 (1.538)	0.286	
Minor complications (any)	31 (6.212)	35 (6.098)	46 (7.438)	44 (7.229)	60 (8.615)	0.278	
Procedure-related death (intra-, post-procedural)	1 (0.200)	1 (0.174)	1 (0.165)	2 (0.344)	1 (0.154)	0.401	
Indication-related death (intra-, post-procedural	1 (0.200)	0 (0.00)	0 (0.00)	1 (0.172)	0 (0.00)	0.485	
Partial radiographic success (remained tip or <4 cm lead fragment)	13 (2.605)	18 (3.136)	22 (3.636)	18 (3.098)	34 (5.231)	0.203	
Complete clinical success	492 (98.60)	563 (98.08)	592 (97.85)	570 (98.11)	634 (97.54)	0.806	
Complete procedural success	481 (96.39)	550 (95.82)	578 (95.54)	556 (95.70)	611 (94.00)	0.322	
Organizational model of TLE procedure. TEE monitoring							
Routine TEE monitoring of lead extraction	261 (52.31)	266 (46.34)	263 (43.37)	263 (45.27)	233 (35.85)	<0.001	<0.001
TLE-related TV dysfunction							
Increase in TR by 1 degree	22 (4.409)	26 (4.530)	29 (4.793)	38 (6.540)	39 (6.000)	0.234	

Table 4. Cont.

	No Stenosis 1	Mild Stenosis 2	Moderate Stenosis 3	Severe Stenosis 4	Total Occlusion 5	ANOVA Kruskal–Wallis Test (1–5) p	ANOVA Kruskal–Wallis Test (1–2) vs. (4–5)
Number of Patients	N = 499	N = 574	N = 605	N = 581	N = 650		
	Mean ± SD n (%)	Mean ± SD n (%)	Mean ± SD n (%)	Mean ± SD n (%)	Mean ± SD n (%)		
Increase in TR by 2 degrees	8 (1.603)	5 (0.871)	13 (2.149)	10 (1.721)	11 (1.692)	0.632	
Increase in TR by 3 degrees	2 (0.401)	2 (0.348)	3 (0.496)	0 (0.00)	3 (0.462)	0.892	
Increase in TR by 2 degrees and to Grade IV	2 (0.401)	4 (0.697)	3 (0.496)	5 (0.861)	3 (0.462)	0.839	
Damage to chordae tendineae during TLE	14 (2.806)	15 (2.613)	18 (2.975)	24 (4.131)	25 (3.846)	0.531	
Short-, mid- and long-term mortality after TLE							
Survival in 1712 ± 1187 (1–4638) days of follow up	375 (75.15)	389 (67.77)	436 (72.07)	373 (64.20)	409 (62.92)	<0.001	<0.001
Death within 48 h	3/499 (0.601)	1/574 (0.174)	1/605 (0.165)	3/581 (0.516)	2/650 (0.308)	0.794	
One-month mortality; 2–30 days; n (% of patients with follow-up longer than 2 days)	4/495 (0.808)	9/573 (1.571)	5/604 (0.828)	4/578 (0.692)	7/648 (1.080)	0.464	
One-year mortality (31–365 days); n (% of patients with follow-up >30 days)	31/491 (6.314)	40/558 (7.168)	43/597 (7.203)	38/573 (6.632)	37/640 (5.781)	0.889	
Three-year mortality (366–1095 days); n (% of patients with follow-up >365 days)	24/433 (5.543)	51/482 (10.581)	50/514 (9.728)	74/499 (14.83)	59/579 (10.19)	<0.001	<0.001
Death at >3 years (at 1095 days); n (% of patients with follow-up >1095 days)	62/359 (17.27)	84/429 (19.58)	70/447 (18.57)	89/447 (19.91)	136/569 (23.90)	<0.001	<0.001

TEE—transesophageal echocardiography, TLE—transvenous lead extraction TR—tricuspid valve regurgitation, TV—tricuspid valve.

Analysis of TLE complexity and degree of LRVSO showed that procedure duration (sheath-to-sheath), extraction of non-functional superfluous leads, occurrence of any technical problem during TLE, lead-to-lead binding, lead fracture during extraction, need to change venous approach, coincidence of three or more technical problems and necessity of using metal sheaths and lasso catheters/snares were associated with the presence of LRVSO (Table 3).

The occurrence of any major complication, urgent rescue cardiac surgery, partial radiographic success (remained tip or <4 cm lead fragment), damage to chordae tendineae, other forms of TLE-related TV dysfunction/damage, complete clinical success and complete procedural success as well as procedure-related death (intra-, post-procedural) did not show any relationship with LRVSO, similar to mortality in the first day, first month and first year after TLE. In contrast, mortality at more than one-year follow-up was significantly higher among patients with severe venous stenosis and complete venous occlusion (Table 4).

Analysis of mortality using the Kaplan–Meier curve confirmed the relationship between LRVSO and long-term survival after TLE (Figure 1).

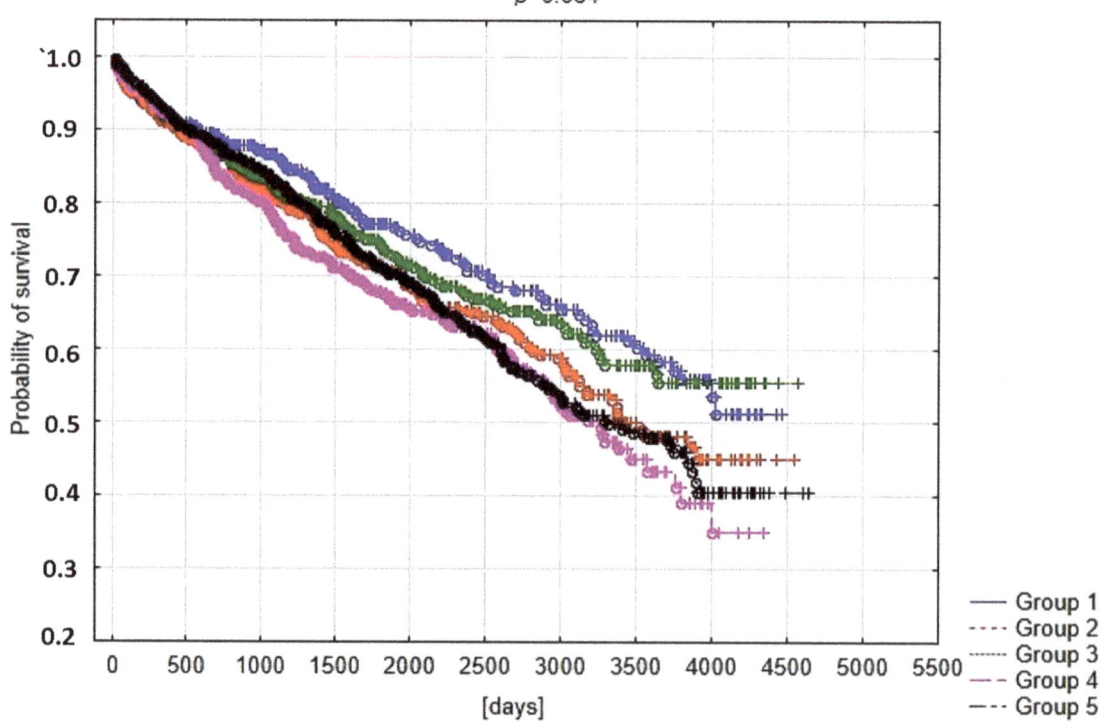

Figure 1. Probability of survival of patients undergoing TLE depending on the degree of LRVSO.

4. Discussion

Venous obstruction is a well-known complication after implantation of a permanent transvenous pacemaker. The incidence of venous obstruction reaches 30–45% with complete occlusion rates of 12% on average and 1–3% for symptomatic occlusion [1–20]. In the current study, severe venous obstruction was identified in 19.94% (40.77% if moderate occlusion was included) whereas complete occlusion in 22.34% of patients. The higher incidence rate of total occlusion in the present study may be a result of long implant duration: cumulative dwell time of the extracted leads was 15.31 ± 12,925 years. Closer evaluation of the clinical factors showed that LVRSO was more common in elderly males with a higher Charlson comorbidity index. Several investigators confirm the contribution of various clinical factors to the occurrence of venous complications [4–6], others show no association between LRVSO and the clinical condition of the patient [7,11]. Analysis of the system/procedure-related factors in the present study demonstrated that the number of extracted leads, lead extraction on the left side or both sides of the chest, extraction of the lead with redundant loop in the heart, extraction of abandoned leads, extraction of leads with long implant duration and a higher risk of MC estimated using the SAFeTY TLE calculator [26] were related to the presence of severe venous stenosis or total venous occlusion. LRVSO was also more common in patients with CRT, having leads with their proximal end in the CVS and a higher number of CIED-related procedures before lead extraction. A similar relationship, especially between the number of extracted leads/long implant duration and LRVSO has been shown in previous reports [5,11].

Out of 20 reports, only four described LRVSO diagnosed just before the TLE procedure [2,6,13,14], and only two assessed the influence of LRVSO on the complexity of TLE [2,6]. The last two studies provide contradicting results. Li et al. in a study of 202 patients concluded that the presence of LRVSO made it more difficult to extract the leads, requiring advanced tools and more time [2]. In contrast, Boczar et al. in a group of 133 pts demonstrated that LRVSO did not influence the effectiveness, safety, and the use of additional tools during TLE procedures [6]. In the present study, the indicators of procedural difficulty and complexity such as procedure duration, extraction of superfluous leads, occurrence of any technical problem, lead-to-lead binding, fracture of the extracted lead, need to change venous approach, coincidence of three or more so-called technical problems and need to use metal sheaths or lasso catheters were related to the presence of LRVSO. The occurrence of any major complication was insignificantly higher in groups with LRVSO as compared to groups without significant stenosis: 2.754 and 2.461% vs. 1.603% and 1.742%, respectively. The need to perform urgent rescue cardiac surgery, partial radiographic success and damage to chordae tendinae during TLE were not significantly associated with the degree of LRVSO. The occurrence of TLE-related TV damage, achievement of complete clinical success and complete procedural success as well as procedure-related death (intra-, post-procedural) were unrelated to LRVSO, similar to mortality in the first day, first month and first year after TLE. This study, however demonstrated a link between TLE difficulty/complexity and the degree of LRVSO, which may be a reflection of implant duration and the total number of extracted leads. Thus, the real problem is only with implantation of new lead (s) because of lead dysfunction or necessity of upgrading the CIED system.

The pathophysiology of LRVSO is not well understood. It is likely that lead-related endothelial trauma incites an inflammatory response of the vessel wall with subsequent thrombosis and scarring. Early (days, weeks) LRVSO seems to be a result of thrombosis which can be treated with low-molecular heparin [16–20]. The role of thrombosis in delayed (months) or late (years) LRVSO is less clear. The inflammatory response of the vessel wall probably induces the formation of scar tissue similar to lead adhesion to the vessel and heart structures, observed on the extracted leads and during TEE [33]. The process of natural maturation makes lead-related fibrotic scar harder and harder leading to its mineralization and calcification. It is well-known that scar tissue in the SVC and in the heart makes lead dissection more difficult [34]. However, so far, nobody has considered scar tissue causing LRVSO and scar tissue around the leads detected during TEE/ICS as the same phenomenon. Looking at narrowing or occlusion of implant veins from this viewpoint we can explain the relationship between LRVSO and TLE complexity, difficulty and complications. Lead dissection in scarred veins is more effort-consuming and sometimes requires stronger pulling on the lead to be extracted. It can also explain the mechanism of TV damage during TLE (fortunately rare). It seems to confirm the concept of simultaneous lead traction from above and below during dissection; it can protect both the SVC wall and the TV [35]. Our results seem to confirm the significance of routine venography before TLE and considering LRVSO as still another risk factor for TLE complexity and major complications.

In the present study, worse long-term survival was demonstrated in patients with a higher degree of LRVSO. The reason for the worse survival rate in this group is not clear and is probably related to other factors as well (possibly a higher Charlson index).

5. Study Limitations

Our study has several limitations worth noting. Routine venography before TLE was performed in all patients except those with contraindications, mainly renal failure. For this reason, an interesting patient subpopulation had been excluded from the study. The database was prospectively integrated, but analysis was performed retrospectively. For the purposes of this study, the population of patients was divided into groups according to maximal venous narrowing without taking into account the site of narrowing/occlusion and the length of venous stenosis/occlusion. Therefore, the present analysis of venograms includes maximal venous narrowing but not the volume of the phenomenon (the number of vessels affected). The classification of patients we used in the study not only enabled comparison of our results with the findings of other investigators, but also maximal venous narrowing was considered a practical marker for predicting the usefulness of veins for implantation of a new lead/catheter.

6. Conclusions

The occurrence of significant venous stenosis/occlusion in patients undergoing TLE is related to some clinical factors (age, male gender, high Charlson comorbidity index) and numerous procedure-related factors, especially long implant duration, extraction of leads with redundant loop in the heart, extraction of abandoned leads, presence of leads with proximal end in the coronary sinus vein and a higher number of CIED-related procedures before lead extraction. LRVSO can be considered as an additional risk factor for TLE complexity. Further research is required to provide evidence for the relationship between scar tissue density encapsulating the leads visible in TEE and the degree of LRVSO. Lead-related venous stenosis/occlusion has no influence on mortality at one-year follow-up, but the presence of severe forms of LRVSO is associated with worse prognosis of patients undergoing TLE at more than one-year follow-up.

Author Contributions: Writing—original draft preparation, M.C.; methodology and statistical study, W.J.; investigation and corresponding author, A.P.; data curation, J.K., D.N., Ł.T. and P.S.; writing-review and editing, A.K. All authors have read and agreed to the published version of the manuscript.

Funding: This research received no external funding.

Institutional Review Board Statement: The study was conducted according to the guidelines of the Declaration of Helsinki, and approved by the of Bioethics Committee at the Regional Medical Chamber in Lublin protocol number 288/2018/KB/VII.

Informed Consent Statement: Informed consent was obtained from all subjects involved in the study.

Data Availability Statement: Readers can access the data supporting the conclusions of the study at www.usuwanieelektrod.pl (accessed on 11 September 2021).

Conflicts of Interest: The authors declare no conflict of interest.

Abbreviations

AnV	innominate (brachiocephalic) vein
AxV	axillary vein
CIED	cardiac implantable electronic device
CRT	cardiac resynchronization therapy
EF	ejection fraction

FU	follow-up
ICD	implantable cardioverter-defibrillator
IVC	inferior vena cava
LR	lead-related
LRVSO	lead-related venous stenosis/occlusion
LV	left ventricle
LVEF	left ventricular ejection fraction
NYHA	The New York Heart Association (functional class)
Pts	patients
PM	pacemaker
RA	right atrium
RV	right ventricle
TEE	transesophageal echocardiography
TLE	transvenous lead extraction
ScV	subclavian vein
SVC	superior vena cava
TV	tricuspid valve
VSO	venous stenosis/occlusion

References

1. Da Costa, S.S.; Scalabrini, N.A.; Costa, R.; Caldas, J.G.; Martinelli, F.M. Incidence and risk factors of upper extremity deep vein lesions after permanent transvenous pacemaker implant: A 6-month follow-up prospective study. *Pacing Clin. Electrophysiol.* 2002, 25, 1301–1306. [CrossRef]
2. Li, X.; Ze, F.; Wang, L.; Li, D.; Duan, J.; Guo, F.; Yuan, C.; Li, Y.; Guo, J. Prevalence of venous occlusion in patients referred for lead extraction: Implications for tool selection. *Europace* 2014, 16, 1795–1799. [CrossRef] [PubMed]
3. Korkeila, P.; Mustonen, P.; Koistinen, J.; Nyman, K.; Ylitalo, A.; Karjalainen, P.; Lund, J.; Airaksinen, J. Clinical and laboratory risk factors of thrombotic complications after pacemaker implantation: A prospective study. *Europace* 2010, 12, 817–824. [CrossRef] [PubMed]
4. Korkeila, P.; Nyman, K.; Ylitalo, A.; Koistinen, J.; Karjalainen, P.; Lund, J.; Airaksinen, K.E. Venous obstruction after pacemaker implantation. *Pacing Clin. Electrophysiol.* 2007, 30, 199–206. [CrossRef] [PubMed]
5. van Rooden, C.J.; Molhoek, S.G.; Rosendaal, F.R.; Schalij, M.J.; Meinders, A.E.; Huisman, M.V. Incidence and risk factors of early venous thrombosis associated with permanent pacemaker leads. *J. Cardiovasc. Electrophysiol.* 2004, 15, 1258–1262. [CrossRef] [PubMed]
6. Boczar, K.; Zabek, A.; Haberka, K.; Debski, M.; Rydlewska, A.; Musial, R.; Lelakowski, J.; Malecka, B. Venous stenosis and occlusion in the presence of endocardial leads in patients referred for transvenous lead extraction. *Acta Cardiol.* 2017, 72, 61–67. [CrossRef]
7. Oginosawa, Y.; Abe, H.; Nakashima, Y. The incidence and risk factors for venous obstruction after implantation of transvenous pacing leads. *Pacing Clin. Electrophysiol.* 2002, 25, 1605–1611. [CrossRef] [PubMed]
8. Crook, B.R.; Gishen, P.; Robinson, C.R.; Oram, S. Occlusion of the subclavian vein associated with cephalic vein pacemaker electrodes. *J. Br. Surg.* 1977, 64, 329–331. [CrossRef]
9. Lickfett, L.; Bitzen, A.; Arepally, A.; Nasir, K.; Wolpert, C.; Jeong, K.M.; Krause, U.; Schimpf, R.; Lewalter, T.; Calkins, H.; et al. Incidence of venous obstruction following insertion of an implantable cardioverter defibrillator. A study of systematic contrast venography on patients presenting for their first elective ICD generator replacement. *EP Eur.* 2004, 6, 25–31. [CrossRef]
10. Goto, Y.; Abe, T.; Sekine, S.; Sakurada, T. Long-term thrombosis after transvenous permanent pacemaker implantation. *Pacing Clin. Electrophysiol.* 1998, 21, 1192–1195. [CrossRef]
11. Haghjoo, M.; Nikoo, M.H.; Fazelifar, A.F.; Alizadeh, A.; Emkanjoo, Z.; Sadr-Ameli, M.A. Predictors of venous obstruction following pacemaker or implantable cardioverter-defibrillator implantation: A contrast venographic study on 100 patients admitted for generator change, lead revision, or device upgrade. *Europace* 2007, 9, 328–332. [CrossRef]
12. Albertini, C.M.M.; Silva, K.R.D.; Leal Filho, J.M.D.M.; Crevelari, E.S.; Martinelli Filho, M.; Carnevale, F.C.; Costa, R. Usefulness of preoperative venography in patients with cardiac implantable electronic devices submitted to lead replacement or device upgrade procedures. *Arq. Bras. Cardiol.* 2018, 111, 686–696. [CrossRef] [PubMed]
13. Bracke, F.; Meijer, A.; Van Gelder, B. Venous occlusion of the access vein in patients referred for lead extraction: Influence of patient and lead characteristics. *Pacing Clin. Electrophysiol.* 2003, 26, 1649–1652. [CrossRef] [PubMed]
14. Sohal, M.; Williams, S.; Akhtar, M.; Shah, A.; Chen, Z.; Wright, M.; O'Neill, M.; Patel, N.; Hamid, S.; Cooklin, M.; et al. Laser lead extraction to facilitate cardiac implantable electronic device upgrade and revision in the presence of central venous obstruction. *Europace* 2014, 16, 81–87. [CrossRef]
15. Figa, F.H.; McCrindle, B.W.; Bigras, J.L.; Hamilton, R.M.; Gow, R.M. Risk factors for venous obstruction in children with transvenous pacing leads. *Pacing Clin. Electrophysiol.* 1997, 20, 1902–1909. [CrossRef] [PubMed]

16. Safi, M.; Akbarzadeh, M.A.; Azinfar, A.; Namazi, M.H.; Khaheshi, I. Upper extremity deep venous thrombosis and stenosis after implantation of pacemakers and defibrillators; A prospective study. *Rom. J. Intern. Med.* **2017**, *55*, 139–144. [CrossRef] [PubMed]
17. Zuber, M.; Huber, P.; Fricker, U.; Buser, P.; Jager, K. Assessment of the subclavian vein in patients with transvenous pacemaker leads. *Pacing Clin. Electrophysiol.* **1998**, *21*, 2621–2630. [CrossRef] [PubMed]
18. Antonelli, D.; Turgeman, Y.; Kaveh, Z.; Artoul, S.; Rosenfeld, T. Short-term thrombosis after transvenous permanent pacemaker insertion. *Pacing Clin. Electrophysiol.* **1989**, *12*, 280–282. [CrossRef]
19. Stoney, W.S.; Addlestone, R.B.; Alford, W.C., Jr.; Burrus, G.R.; Frist, R.A.; Thomas, C.S., Jr. The incidence of venous thrombosis following long-term transvenous pacing. *Ann. Thorac. Surg.* **1976**, *22*, 166–170. [CrossRef]
20. Sticherling, C.; Chough, S.P.; Baker, R.L.; Wasmer, K.; Oral, H.; Tada, H.; Horwood, L.; Kim, M.H.; Pelosi, F.; Michaud, G.F.; et al. Prevalence of central venous occlusion in patients with chronic defibrillator leads. *Am. Heart J.* **2001**, *141*, 813–816. [CrossRef]
21. Wilkoff, B.L.; Love, C.J.; Byrd, C.L.; Bongiorni, M.G.; Carrillo, R.G.; Crossley, G.H., 3rd; Epstein, L.M.; Friedman, R.A.; Kennergren, C.E.; Mitkowski, P.; et al. Heart Rhythm Society; American Heart Association. Transvenous lead extraction: Heart Rhythm Society expert consensus on facilities, training, indications, and patient management: This document was endorsed by the American Heart Association (AHA). *Heart Rhythm* **2009**, *6*, 1085–1104. [CrossRef]
22. Kusumoto, F.M.; Schoenfeld, M.H.; Wilkoff, B.; Berul, C.I.; Birgersdotter-Green, U.M.; Carrillo, R.; Cha, Y.M.; Clancy, J.; Deharo, J.C.; Ellenbogen, K.A.; et al. 2017 HRS expert consensus statement on cardiovascular implantable electronic device lead management and extraction. *Heart Rhythm* **2017**, *14*, e503–e551. [CrossRef]
23. Bongiorni, M.G.; Burri, H.; Deharo, J.C.; Starck, C.; Kennergren, C.; Saghy, L.; Rao, A.; Tascini, C.; Lever, N.; Kutarski, A.; et al. 2018 EHRA expert consensus statement on lead extraction: Recommendations on definitions, endpoints, research trial design, and data collection requirements for clinical scientific studies and registries: Endorsed by APHRS/HRS/LAHRS. *EP Eur.* **2018**, *20*, 1217. [CrossRef] [PubMed]
24. Brunner, M.P.; Cronin, E.M.; Wazni, O.; Baranowski, B.; Saliba, W.I.; Sabik, J.F.; Lindsay, B.D.; Wilkoff, B.L.; Tarakji, K.G. Outcomes of patients requiring emergent surgical or endovascular intervention for catastrophic complications during transvenous lead extraction. *Heart Rhythm* **2014**, *11*, 419–425. [CrossRef] [PubMed]
25. Bashir, J.; Fedoruk, L.M.; Ofiesh, J.; Karim, S.S.; Tyers, G.F.O. Classification and Surgical Repair of Injuries Sustained during Transvenous Lead Extraction. *Circ. Arrhythmia Electrophysiol.* **2016**, *9*, e003741. [CrossRef] [PubMed]
26. Jacheć, W.; Polewczyk, A.; Polewczyk, M.; Tomasik, A.; Kutarski, A. Transvenous Lead Extraction SAFeTY Score for Risk Stratification and Proper Patient Selection for Removal Procedures using Mechanical Tools. *J. Clin. Med.* **2020**, *9*, 361. [CrossRef] [PubMed]
27. Sidhu, B.S.; Ayis, S.; Gould, J.; Elliott, M.K.; Mehta, V.; Kennergren, C.; Butter, C.; Deharo, J.C.; Kutarski, A.; Maggioni, A.P.; et al. Risk stratification of patients undergoing transvenous lead extraction with the ELECTRa Registry Outcome Score (EROS). An ESC EHRA EORP European lead extraction ConTRolled ELECTRa registry analysis. *EP Eur.* **2021**, *23*, 1462–1471, Online ahead of print.
28. Kancharla, K.; Acker, N.G.; Li, Z.; Samineni, S.; Cai, C.; Espinosa, R.E.; Osborn, M.; Mulpuru, S.K.; Asirvatham, S.J.; Friedman, P.A.; et al. Efficacy and safety of transvenous lead extraction in the device laboratory and operating room guided by a novel risk stratification scheme. *JACC Clin. Electrophysiol.* **2019**, *5*, 174–182. [CrossRef]
29. Bontempi, L.; Vassanelli, F.; Cerini, M.; D'Aloia, A.; Vizzardi, E.; Gargaro, A.; Chiusso, F.; Mamedouv, R.; Lipari, A.; Curnis, A. Predicting the difficulty of a lead extraction procedure: The LED index. *J. Cardiovasc. Med.* **2014**, *15*, 668–673. [CrossRef]
30. Nowosielecka, D.; Jacheć, W.; Polewczyk, A.; Tułecki, Ł.; Tomków, K.; Stefańczyk, P.; Tomaszewski, A.; Brzozowski, W.; Szcześniak-Stańczyk, D.; Kleinrok, A.; et al. Transesophageal Echocardiography as a Monitoring Tool during Transvenous Lead Extraction-Does It Improve Procedure Effectiveness? *J. Clin. Med.* **2020**, *9*, 1382. [CrossRef]
31. Nowosielecka, D.; Polewczyk, A.; Jacheć, W.; Tułecki, Ł.; Tomków, K.; Stefańczyk, P.; Kleinrok, A.; Kutarski, A. A new approach to the continuous monitoring of transvenous lead extraction using transesophageal echocardiography-Analysis of 936 procedures. *Echocardiography* **2020**, *37*, 601–611. [CrossRef] [PubMed]
32. Nowosielecka, D.; Polewczyk, A.; Jacheć, W.; Kleinrok, A.; Tułecki, Ł.; Kutarski, A. Transesophageal echocardiography for the monitoring of transvenous lead extraction. *Kardiol. Pol. (Pol. Heart J.)* **2020**, *78*, 1206–1214. [CrossRef] [PubMed]
33. Nowosielecka, D.; Polewczyk, A.; Jacheć, W.; Tułecki, Ł.; Kleinrok, A.; Kutarski, A. Echocardiographic findings in patients with cardiac implantable electronic devices-analysis of factors predisposing to lead-associated changes. *Clin. Physiol. Funct. Imaging* **2021**, *41*, 25–41. [CrossRef] [PubMed]
34. Nowosielecka, D.; Jacheć, W.; Polewczyk, A.; Tułecki, Ł.; Kleinrok, A.; Kutarski, A. Prognostic Value of Preoperative Echocardiographic Findings in Patients Undergoing Transvenous Lead Extraction. *Int. J. Environ. Res. Public Health* **2021**, *18*, 1862. [CrossRef] [PubMed]
35. Schaller, R.D.; Sadek, M.M.; Cooper, J.M. Simultaneous lead traction from above and below: A novel technique to reduce the risk of superior vena cava injury during transvenous lead extraction. *Heart Rhythm* **2018**, *15*, 1655–1663. [CrossRef]

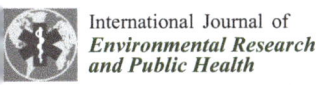

Case Report

Successful Catheter Ablation of the "R on T" Ventricular Fibrillation

Zofia Lasocka, Alicja Dąbrowska-Kugacka *, Ewa Lewicka, Aleksandra Liżewska-Springer and Tomasz Królak

Department of Cardiology and Electrotherapy, Medical University of Gdańsk, 80-211 Gdansk, Poland; zofia.lasocka@gumed.edu.pl (Z.L.); ewa.lewicka@gumed.edu.pl (E.L.); aleksandra.lizewska-springer@gumed.edu.pl (A.L.-S.); tomasz.krolak@gumed.edu.pl (T.K.)
* Correspondence: alicja.dabrowska-kugacka@gumed.edu.pl

Abstract: In patients with idiopathic ventricular fibrillation (VF), recurrent implantable cardioverter-defibrillator (ICD) shocks might increase mortality risk and reduce patients' quality of life. Catheter ablation of triggering ectopic beats is considered to be an effective method. We present a patient with recurrent VF, caused by the "R on T" premature ventricular complexes. In the presented case radiofrequency catheter ablation efficiently eliminated arrhythmia trigger, which was possible to detect thanks to the intracardiac electrocardiograms (ECG's) stored in the ICD.

Keywords: ventricular fibrillation; R on T phenomenon; catheter ablation; mapping

1. Introduction

Idiopathic ventricular fibrillation (VF) occurs in healthy individuals without structural heart disease. Although most sudden cardiac deaths (SCDs) are associated with identifiable causes, idiopathic VF accounts for 5% to 10% of out-of-hospital cardiac arrest [1]. In such patients, the gold standard treatment for either primary or secondary prevention of VF is the insertion of an implantable cardioverter-defibrillator (ICD). The goal is however to determine the mechanism of spontaneous arrhythmia. Intracardiac electrocardiograms (IECGs) stored in ICD provide information about cardiac rhythm preceding arrhythmic events and may be helpful to reveal their mechanism [2].

Mapping during VF reveals few sources triggering the arrhythmia. In patients with idiopathic VF, premature ventricular complexes (PVCs) triggers usually arise either from right ventricular outflow tract region or from the Purkinje network [3]. The Purkinje network fibers originate from the bundle branches, whose function is to distribute the depolarization wavefront to the left and right ventricles, allowing for their simultaneous activation. However, Purkinje cells have shown to have abnormal automaticity and triggered activity, what may play a significant role in the initiation of VF in patients with both structural heart disease and normal hearts [4–6].

As recurrent ICD shocks might increase mortality risk and reduce patients' quality of life, anti-arrhythmic drugs are recommended [7]. According to the Optimal Pharmacological Therapy in Cardioverter Defibrillator Patients (OPTIC) trial, which included patients with secondary prevention ICD indication, amiodarone compared to b-blocker reduced the risk of both appropriate and inappropriate shocks [8]. However, if pharmacological treatment is not successful or the patient experiences drug-related side effects, radiofrequency (RF) ablation can be considered if VF is triggered by PVCs [3–5].

2. Case Report

We present the history of a 62-year-old male with recurrent VF triggered by the "R on T" ventricular premature beats. In 2006, he underwent cardiac arrest and was diagnosed with idiopathic VF, as no apparent structural cardiac disease or other cause of the arrhythmia was found. Twelve-lead surface electrocardiogram (ECG) showed sinus rhythm, with normal QRS complexes and repolarization, while 24-hour ECG monitoring revealed multiple monomorphic PVCs (<1000) and no other abnormalities. In the echocardiographic

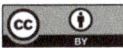

examination good left ventricular ejection fraction (LVEF) of 70%, without any segmental hypo/akinesis was found. A coronary angiogram revealed no narrowing in the coronary arteries. Cardiac magnetic resonance was not performed in 2006, as it was not widely available at that time. The patient was implanted with a single-chamber ICD for secondary prevention of sudden cardiac death. At hospital discharge, anti-arrhythmic treatment with amiodarone 200 mg and metoprolol 50 mg daily was prescribed.

Within the next year, amiodarone was withheld due to thyreotoxicosis. Thyroid function was normalized, metoprolol dose was increased to 175 mg daily, but VF episodes occurred about one to two times per year and were terminated by ICD shock. As presented on Figure 1, the 12-lead ECG revealed singular PVCs with morphology of right ventricular free wall origin. The initial ICD was replaced in 2016 due to battery replacement indications. Stored IECGs revealed VF episodes initiated by the "R on T" PVCs and terminated spontaneously, by anti-tachycardia pacing (ATP) or high-voltage shocks (Figure 2A,B). To reduce the number of painful ICD interventions, as pharmacological treatment was not efficient, the patient was referred for elective electrophysiological study (EPS) and RF ablation of ectopic beats. Pre-ablation 24-hour ECG monitoring showed sinus rhythm, 1629 single monomorphic PVCs with around 300 qualified as "R on T".

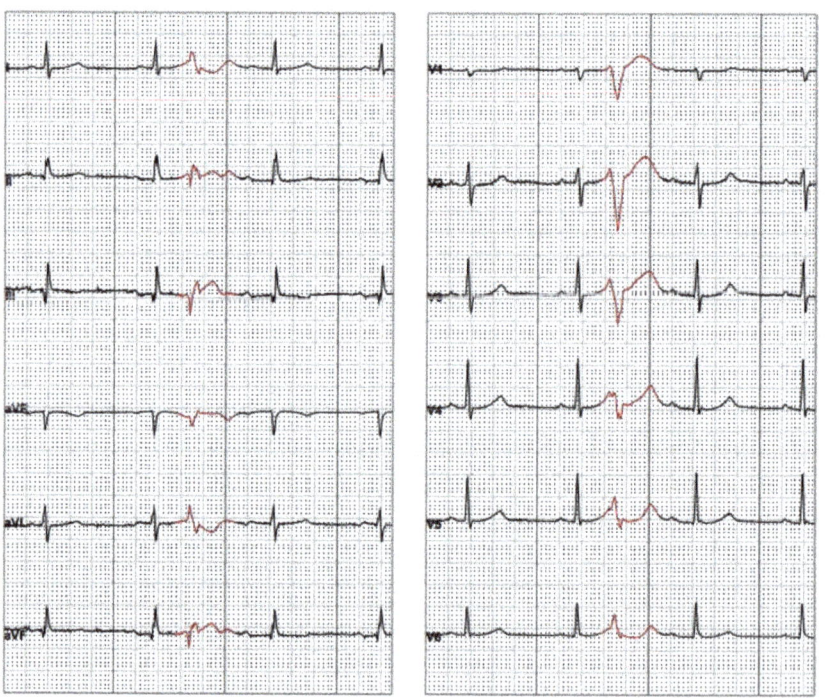

Figure 1. 12-lead electrocardiogram (ECG) with premature ventricular complex (PVC) originating from the right ventricular free wall.

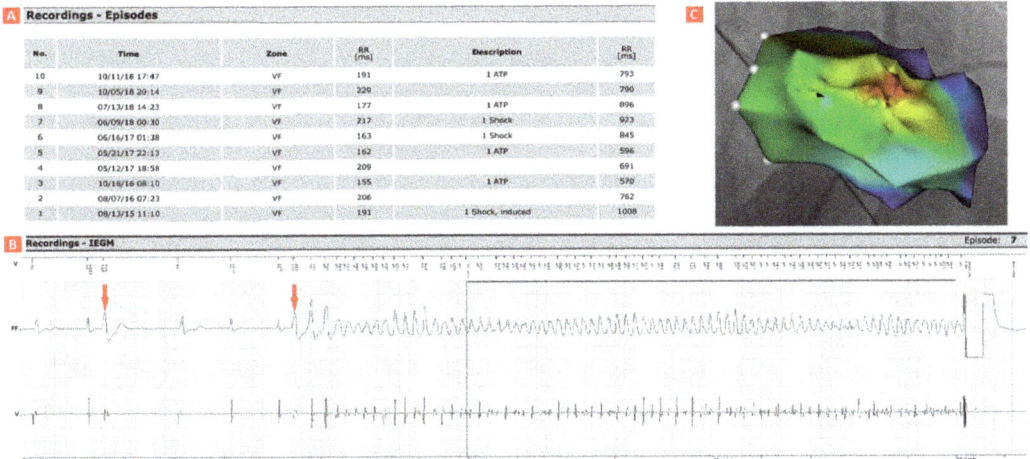

Figure 2. Ventricular fibrillation (VF) episodes resulting in implantable cardioverter-defibrillator (ICD) interventions, from the time of ICD reimplantation to the decision to perform radiofrequency ablation (**A**); ICD intracardiac recording showing the premature ventricular complex (PVC) triggering VF. VF initiating PVC is similar to the previously registered PVC (arrows) (**B**); Right anterior oblique 30° view of right ventricular endocardial activation map obtained during spontaneous PVCs: the earliest activation site was located in the antero-lateral right ventricular free wall (red area) (**C**). ATP—antitachycardia pacing, IEGM—intracardiac electrocardiogram, RR—consecutive R waves on the IEGM.

Ablation catheter (Thermocool Smarttouch SF, Biosense Webster, Johnson and Johnson Medical, Ltd., Irvine, CA, USA) was introduced to the right ventricle through a femoral approach under fluoroscopic guidance. Using CARTO 3 mapping system (version 7.1, Biosense Webster, Irvine, CA, USA) three types of right ventricular endocardial maps were created: the bipolar map during sinus rhythm, the correlation map of pace-mapping (using PaSo module), the activation map during clinical PVCs. The bipolar map revealed no abnormalities. The earliest endocardial activation site and maximal pace-mapping correlation (93% according to PaSo module) was found in the antero-lateral right ventricular free wall (Figure 2C). RF ablation current was delivered at 30 W of power-controlled mode with a temperature of 43 °C for 30–60 sec. Clinical spontaneous PVCs were eliminated, but pacing delivered from right ventricular lead of ICD occasionally induced single PVCs with slightly different morphology compared to the clinical PVCs.

In the follow-up, until June 2021 the patient remained asymptomatic and without episodes of VF or ventricular tachycardia in the ICD control. The patient's quality of life increased significantly. 24-hours ECG monitoring revealed sinus rhythm and only eight PVCs. Metoprolol was gradually reduced to 50 mg daily.

3. Discussion

Our case demonstrates the efficacy of RF ablation in a patient with recurrent idiopathic VF, and ineffective antiarrhythmic treatment. IECGs from the ICD provided information about the mechanism of the arrhythmic episodes, which in the presented case was the "R on T" phenomenon. Indeed, electrocardiogram stored in the ICD devices is comparable to continuous Holter monitoring. Information, such as the day and time of the episode, the preceding heart rate, the influence of preceding premature beats and their morphology can be obtained from the IECG records analysis. In other words, it enables the physician to identify the arrhythmia trigger, underlying recurrent VF or ventricular tachycardia, and consequently, to apply the most appropriate treatment [2].

In up to 70% of patients after ICD implantation antiarrhythmic agents need to be initiated, in order to treat atrial tachyarrhythmias, terminate ventricular arrhythmias and decrease the frequency of ICD shocks. Class III antiarrhythmic drugs, such as amiodarone and sotalol, are widely considered to be effective in preventing ICD shocks [9]. However, potential cardiac and drug-related adverse effects of antiarrhythmics should be taken into consideration, as apart from ICD/drug interactions, these are the most frequent causes of drug discontinuation. In our case amiodarone was withheld due to thyreotoxicosis. The concomitant pharmacological therapy turned out insufficient to prevent recurrent ventricular tachyarrhythmias.

To reduce the number of ICD shocks, catheter ablation of the triggering PVCs was recommended. Pace-mapping allowed identification of the PVCs' origin. According to recent reports, PVCs triggering VF arise either from the myocardium (right or left ventricular outflow tract) or from the distal Purkinje network [4]. In the study on 27 patients with recurrent episodes of idiopathic VF, PVCs originated from the Purkinje conducting system in 23 patients, while from right ventricular outflow tract only in 4 study counterparts [3]. There is a growing body of evidence that the Purkinje network, consisting of a single branch on the right and 2 larger branches on the left heart side, plays a significant role in both the initiation and maintenance of VF. It has been proved that RF ablation of arrhythmia triggers effectively prevent VF recurrence in a high-risk population [5,6]. Decreasing the incidence of ventricular arrhythmias catheter ablation may reduce defibrillation requirement and improve the patient's quality of life.

4. Conclusions

In conclusion, implantation of ICD is the gold standard treatment for both primary and secondary prevention of SCD. The primary goal is to identify the mechanism underlying the spontaneous arrhythmia. In the presented case, RF ablation efficiently eliminated the arrhythmia trigger, which was identified thanks to the stored intracardiac electrograms. RF ablation is considered an effective method of arrhythmia termination, in case of antiarrhythmic drugs intolerance or inappropriate ICD shocks. Although the long-term results are very encouraging, ablation of triggering PVCs for VF does not replace ICD implantation.

Author Contributions: Conceptualization, A.D.-K.; formal analysis, Z.L., A.D.-K., E.L., and T.K.; investigation, Z.L., A.D.-K., and E.L.; writing—original draft preparation, Z.L.; writing—review and editing, A.D.-K., E.L., A.L.-S., and T.K.; supervision, A.D.-K., E.L. All authors have read and agreed to the published version of the manuscript.

Funding: This research received no external funding.

Institutional Review Board Statement: The study was conducted according to the guidelines of the Declaration of Helsinki, and approved by the Independent Bioethics Committee for Scientific Research at Medical University of Gdansk–NKBBN/660/2021.

Informed Consent Statement: Written informed consent has been obtained from the patient to publish this paper.

Conflicts of Interest: The authors declare no conflict of interest.

References

1. Belhassen, B.; Viskin, S. Idiopathic ventricular tachycardia and fibrillation. *J. Cardiovasc. Electrophysiol.* **1993**, *4*, 356–368. [CrossRef] [PubMed]
2. Auricchio, A.; Hartung, W.; Geller, C.; Klein, H. Clinical relevance of stored electrograms for implantable cardioverter-defibrillator (ICD) troubleshooting and understanding of mechanisms for ventricular tachyarrhythmias. *Am. J. Cardiol.* **1996**, *78*, 33–41. [CrossRef]
3. Haïssaguerre, M.; Shoda, M.; Jaïs, P.; Nogami, A.; Shah, D.C.; Kautzner, J.; Arentz, T.; Kalushe, D.; Lamaison, D.; Griffith, M.; et al. Mapping and ablation of idiopathic ventricular fibrillation. *Circulation* **2002**, *106*, 962–967. [CrossRef] [PubMed]
4. Gianni, C.; Burkhardt, J.D.; Trivedi, C.; Mohanty, S.; Natale, A. The role of the Purkinje network in premature ventricular complex-triggered ventricular fibrillation. *J. Interv. Card Electrophysiol.* **2018**, *52*, 375–383. [CrossRef] [PubMed]
5. Knecht, S.; Sacher, F.; Wright, M.; Hocini, M.; Nogami, A.; Arentz, T.; Petit, B.; Franck, R.; De Chillou, C.; Lamaison, D.; et al. Long-term follow-up of idiopathic ventricular fibrillation ablation: A multicenter study. *J. Am. Coll. Cardiol.* **2009**, *54*, 522–528. [CrossRef] [PubMed]

6. Haïssaguerre, M.; Duchateau, J.; Dubois, R.; Hocini, M.; Cheniti, G.; Sacher, F.; Lavergne, T.; Probst, V.; Surget, E.; Vigmond, E.; et al. Idiopathic Ventricular Fibrillation: Role of Purkinje System and Microstructural Myocardial Abnormalities. *JACC Clin. Electrophysiol.* **2020**, *6*, 591–608. [CrossRef] [PubMed]
7. Larsen, G.K.; Evans, J.; Lambert, W.E.; Chen, Y.; Raitt, M.H. Shocks burden and increased mortality in implantable cardioverter-defibrillator patients. *Heart Rhythm.* **2011**, *8*, 1881–1886. [CrossRef] [PubMed]
8. Hohnloser, S.H.; Dorian, P.; Roberts, R.; Gent, M.; Israel, C.W.; Fain, E.; Champagne, J.; Connolly, S.J. Effect of amiodarone and sotalol on ventricular defibrillation threshold: The optimal pharmacological therapy in cardioverter defibrillator patients (OPTIC) trial. *Circulation* **2006**, *114*, 104–109. [CrossRef] [PubMed]
9. Van Herendael, H.; Pinter, A.; Ahmad, K.; Korley, V.; Mangat, I.; Dorian, P. Role of antiarrhythmic drugs in patients with implantable cardioverter defibrillators. *Europace* **2010**, *12*, 618–625. [CrossRef] [PubMed]

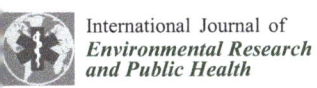

Article

Analysis of Risk Factors for Major Complications of 1500 Transvenous Lead Extraction Procedures with Especial Attention to Tricuspid Valve Damage

Łukasz Tułecki [1], Anna Polewczyk [2,3,*], Wojciech Jacheć [4], Dorota Nowosielecka [5], Konrad Tomków [1], Paweł Stefańczyk [5], Jarosław Kosior [6], Krzysztof Duda [7], Maciej Polewczyk [8] and Andrzej Kutarski [9]

1. Department of Cardiac Surgery, The Pope John Paul II Province Hospital of Zamość, 22-400 Zamość, Poland; luke27@poczta.onet.pl (Ł.T.); konradtomkow@wp.pl (K.T.)
2. Department of Physiology, Pathophysiology and Clinical Immunology Collegium Medicum, The Jan Kochanowski University, 25-369 Kielce, Poland
3. Department of Cardiac Surgery, Świętokrzyskie Cardiology Center, 25-369 Kielce, Poland
4. 2nd Department of Cardiology, Silesian Medical University, 41-808 Zabrze, Poland; wjachec@interia.pl
5. Department of Cardiology, The Pope John Paul II Province Hospital of Zamość, 22-400 Zamość, Poland; dornowos@wp.pl (D.N.); paolost@interia.pl (P.S.)
6. Department of Cardiology, Masovian Specialist Hospital of Radom, 26-617 Radom, Poland; jaroslaw.kosior@icloud.com
7. Department of Cardiac Surgery, Masovian Specialist Hospital of Radom, 26-617 Radom, Poland; kadeder@gmail.com
8. Faculty of Medicine and Health Studies, Jan Kochanowski University, 25-369 Kielce, Poland; Maciek.polewczyk@gmail.com
9. Department of Cardiology, Medical University of Lublin, 20-509 Lublin, Poland; a_kutarski@yahoo.com
* Correspondence: annapolewczyk@wp.pl

Abstract: Background: Transvenous lead extraction (TLE) is a relatively safe procedure, but it may cause severe complications such as cardiac/vascular wall tear (CVWT) and tricuspid valve damage (TVD). Methods: The risk factors for CVWT and TVD were examined based on an analysis of data of 1500 extraction procedures performed in two high-volume centers. Results: The total number of major complications was 33 (2.2%) and included 22 (1.5%) CVWT and 12 (0.8%) TVD (with one case of combined complication). Patients with hemorrhagic complications were younger, more often women, less often presenting low left ventricular ejection fraction (LVEF) and those who received their first cardiac implantable electronic device (CIED) earlier than the control group. A typical patient with CVWT was a pacemaker carrier, having more leads (including abandoned leads and excessive loops) with long implant duration and a history of multiple CIED-related procedures. The risk factors for TVD were similar to those for CVWT, but the patients were older and received their CIED about nine years earlier. Any form of tissue scar and technical problems were much more common in the two groups of patients with major complications. Conclusions: The risk factors for CVWT and TVD are similar, and the most important ones are related to long lead dwell time and its consequences for the heart (various forms of fibrotic scarring). The occurrence of procedural complications does not affect long-term survival in patients undergoing lead extraction.

Keywords: transvenous lead extraction; lead extraction-related major complications; cardiac/vascular wall tear; worsening tricuspid regurgitation

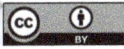

1. Introduction

Transvenous lead extraction (TLE) is now an integral part of the lead management strategy [1–5]. Fibrotic scarring around the leads [6] places the patient at risk of fatal complications such as venous or cardiac injury with severe bleeding [7–11] or worsening tricuspid regurgitation [12–18]. The problem of tricuspid valve damage was overlooked in several previous guideline revisions [1–4] and addressed only in the recent ones [4,5].

Up to date, several attempts have been made in search of the risk factors predictive of major complications [19–22]. Such knowledge is useful to plan the strategy of TLE including selection of the center, venue, first operator, organizational model (staging of safety precautions). Analysis of the well-and lesser-known factors facilitates the calculation of the real risk of major complications [23–27]. It also helps better prepare and provide preoperative information to the patient and family members. However, most of the available risk calculators had been invented, when worsening tricuspid regurgitation was not accepted officially as major complication of lead removal (before 2017). Recently, more and more investigators have paid attention to inadvertent tricuspid valve damage during TLE [12–18], and an analysis of risk factors that are specifically associated with this complication seems to be justified. Their identification, especially a history of pacing and previous lead management strategies may change our current routine and update the guidelines in the future.

The aim of this study was to determine circumstances of occurrence and risk factors (patient-dependent, pacing history-related, procedure-related) of cardiac/vascular wall tear (CVWT) and TV damage (TVD) considered as TLE major complication with focus on the utility of information obtained in monitoring by transesophageal echocardiography (TEE) during lead extraction.

2. Materials and Methods

This study was a post-hoc analysis of the clinical data of 1500 patients undergoing transvenous lead extraction at two high-volume centers between June 2015 and April 2021. We compared the clinical and procedure-related factors as well as echocardiographic findings in patients with major complications during lead extraction (with particular emphasis on cardiac/vascular wall damage and tricuspid valve damage) and in individuals without TLE-related complications.

The following clinical variables were taken into account: age, gender, NYHA class, renal failure and infectious indications for TLE. The procedure-related variables included type of the implanted system, the number and type of leads being extracted, as well as the risk for the occurrence of major complications measured as the SAFeTY TLE score [23]. The echocardiographic variables considered for the analysis included left ventricular ejection fraction (LVEF), the degree of tricuspid valve (TV) dysfunction before and after TLE, mean right ventricular systolic pressure (RVSP), the presence of fibrotic scarring, lead thickening, lead-to-lead binding, lead adherence to any heart structure and right ventricular wall perforation by the lead. The study subgroups were also compared with regard to the course of the procedure measuring TLE duration time (skin-to-skin and sheath-to-sheath duration), presence of lead-to-lead adhesions, occurrence of any technical problem during TLE, block at lead venous entry site, extracted lead fracture, Byrd dilator torsion/collapse, utility of specific tools such as Evolution, TightRail, lasso catheters/snares and need for temporary pacing during the procedure. Of the echocardiographic and hemodynamic monitoring parameters we compared pulling on the cardiac walls and other leads as well as a drop in blood pressure during TLE. This study also analyzed complete procedural and clinical success as well as short-and long-term survival (mortality at 1 month, 1 year, 3 years and >3 years after TLE).

2.1. Lead Extraction Procedure

Lead extraction procedure was defined according to the most recent guidelines on the management of lead-related complications (HRS 2017 and EHRA 2018) [2–5]. Indications for TLE and type of periprocedural complications were defined according to the 2017 HRS Expert Consensus Statement on Cardiovascular Implantable Electronic Device Lead Management and Extraction [4].

Most procedures were performed using nonpowered mechanical systems such as Byrd polypropylene dilator sheaths (Cook® Medical, Leechburg, PA, USA), if only possible via the implant vein. If technical difficulties arose, alternative venous approaches or additional tools such as Evolution (Cook® Medical, Leechburg, PA, USA), TightRail (Spectranetix, Sunnyvale, CA, USA), lassos, basket catheters were utilized. The excimer laser was not applied.

All extraction procedures were performed following the same organizational model in accordance with the current guidelines. The operating team consisted of a very experienced extractor, cardiac surgeon, anesthesiologist and echocardiographist. The procedures were performed in a hybrid room or a cardiac surgery operating room, with a full range of equipment for an emergency rescue.

The SAFeTY TLE score was used to assess the risk for the occurrence of major complications related to TLE [23] using an online calculator, available at http://alamay2.linuxpl.info/kalkulator/ (accessed on 27 August 2021). The calculator is available on the website www.usuwanieelektro.pl. (accessed on 27 August 2021).

The following terms were used to assess the duration of the procedure: skin-to-skin time and sheath-to-sheath time. The skin-to-skin time is time in minutes from the cutting to the sewing of the skin. It includes not only dissection of the lead (s), but also lead re-implantation for non-infectious indications. The sheath-to-sheath time (in minutes) is total time for dissection and removal of all scheduled leads.

2.2. TEE Monitoring during TLE

Transthoracic examinations (TTE) and transesophageal echocardiography monitoring were performed using Philips iE33 or GE Vivid S 70 machines equipped with X7-2t Live 3D or 6VT-D probes. All recordings were archived and, in accordance with the guidelines, included a preoperative examination, navigation during TLE, and postoperative evaluation of the effectiveness of the procedure with an assessment of possible complications. [28–31]. The projections and consecutive stages of echocardiographic monitoring were described in detail in previous publications [28–31]. The preoperative monitoring phase (TTE and TEE) included assessment of lead position, lead-to-lead binding and adhesions between the leads and the walls of the heart, the presence of additional masses on the leads, and evaluation of tricuspid valve function.

The intraoperative phase of TEE monitoring allowed visualization of direct pulling on the heart and the right ventricular cavity during lead removal. Often, a drop in blood pressure is observed, and monitoring makes it possible to clarify the cause of this phenomenon [28–31]. Additionally, it is possible to quickly assess damage to the heart wall with accumulation of excess fluid in the pericardial sac [29,30]. The post-procedural phase of TTE and TEE monitoring includes reassessment of cardiac/vascular wall injury and tricuspid valve function, detection of lead remnants and residual vegetations.

2.3. Statistical Analysis

The Shapiro–Wilk test showed that most continuous variables were normally distributed. For uniformity, all continuous variables are presented as the mean ± standard deviation. The categorical variables are presented as number and percentage. The study population was divided into the following groups: A—patients with hemorrhagic complications due to cardiac/vascular wall tear; B—patients with tricuspid valve damage, C—patients from groups A and B, and D—patients without complications. The significance of differences between groups (A, B, C vs. D) was determined using the nonparametric Chi2 test with Yates's correction or the unpaired "U" Mann–Whitney test, as appropriate. The Spearman r correlation was determined for pulling on vascular or cardiac structures during TLE and maximal drop in blood pressure. A p-value less than 0.05 was considered as statistically significant.

Statistical analysis was performed with Statistica version 13.3 (TIBCO Software Inc., Palo Alto, CA, USA).

2.4. Approval of the Bioethics Committee

All patients gave their informed written consent to undergo TLE and to use anonymous data from their medical records, approved by the Bioethics Committee at the Regional Chamber of Physicians in Lublin no. 288/2018/KB/VII. The study was carried out in accordance with the ethical standards of the 1964 Declaration of Helsinki.

3. Results

The study population consisted of 1500 patients, mean age 68.11 years, 39.87% of females. The mean left ventricular ejection fraction (LVEF) was 49.26%, renal failure occurred in 25.00% of patients, the Charlson comorbidity index was 5.10. The indications for lead extraction included systemic infection (with pocket infection or not) in 15.33% of patients, local (pocket) infection in 6.00%, lead failure (replacement) in 57.67%, change of pacing mode/upgrading/downgrading in 7.33%, other in 12.87% of patients. Overall, 67.07% of patients had a pacemaker, 23.93% cardioverter-defibrillator (ICD), and 8.87% resynchronization device (CRT-D). The dwell time of the oldest lead per patient before TLE was 112.1 (months), the cumulative lead dwell time before TLE was 17.01 (years).

Patients with hemorrhagic complications (cardiac/vascular wall tear) were significantly younger and received their first cardiac implantable electronic device (CIED) 15 years earlier than in the control group. There were twice as many women as men, and significantly fewer patients with low LVEF and in NYHA class III or IV. The Charlson comorbidity index was much lower as compared to the control group. The indications for TLE were comparable to the remaining groups of patients (Table 1).

Patients with TV damage (TVD group) were older compared to the other subgroups but received their first CIED nine years earlier. There were fewer women, and similarly to CVWD group, there were fewer patients with low LVEF and in NYHA class III or IV. The Charlson comorbidity index was slightly lower as compared to the control group. The indications for TLE were comparable to CVWD and control groups. TVD patients frequently had an abandoned lead, more CIED-related procedures and more often longer implant duration similar to CVWT patients (Table 1).

The number of extracted leads per patient ($p = 0.056$), the need to extract three or more leads, extraction of leads with redundant loops, extraction of abandoned lead (s) and extraction of atrial leads were regarded as intraprocedural risk factors for CVWT and TVD. There was one exception, however. Atrial lead extraction was strongly associated with CVWT but not with TV damage, and extraction of abandoned leads was more likely to be related to CVWT (Table 2).

Implant duration was the strongest predictor of both CVWT and TVD. An interesting finding was the value of the SAFeTY TLE score estimating the risk of procedure. The calculator had been created before 2017 when TVD was not considered as major complication; it works excellently and the calculated (automatically) risk of CVWT and TVD was 5.2-fold and 3.4-fold higher than in the control group.

Passive fixation leads were also predictors of CVWT and TVD (RAA tear was the most frequent finding) (Table 2).

Preoperative TTE and TEE demonstrated that the state of the tricuspid valve was similar in groups with major complications of TLE. These groups were characterized by higher LVEF and lower RVSP. TEE before TLE provided much more valuable information. Oscillating scar tissue on the leads, lead thickening, lead-to-lead binding, lead adhering to any heart structure, lead adhering to the tricuspid valve, to the walls of the superior vena cava (SVC), right atrium (RA) and right ventricle (RV), the presence of any form of scar tissue were much more often detected in the two groups with major complications. Additionally, all forms of scar tissue were more frequent in patients with postprocedural TVD. However, there was one exception: a small percentage of leads adhering to the RA wall in patients with postprocedural TVD (Table 3).

Table 1. Patient/system/history of pacing.

	Hemorrhagic Complication (Cardiac/Vascular Wall Tear)	Tricuspid Valve Damage	All Major Complications (Mixed Damages 1 Case)	Control Group (No Major Complications)
Groups of patients	A N = 22 (1.5%) Mean ± SD n (%)	B N = 12 (0.8%) Mean ± SD n (%)	C N = 33 (2.2%) Mean ± S n (%)	D N = 1467 Mean ± SD n (%)
		Patients		
Patient age during TLE [years]	63.14 ± 13.91 $p = 0.009$	68.75 ± 21.98 $p = 0.116$	65.82 ± 16.84 $p = 0.005$	68.16 ± 13.96
Patient age at first implantation [years]	45.32 ± 16.98 $p < 0.001$	50.58 ± 26.16 $p = 0.007$	47.97 ± 20.23 $p < 0.001$	59.06 ± 15.58
Sex (% of female patients)	17 (77.30) $p = 0.004$	5 (41.70) $p = 0.979$	21 (63.60) $p = 0.005$	555 (37.80)
NYHA class III & IV (%)	1 (4.50) $p = 0.192$	0 (0.00) $p = 0.227$	1 (3.00) $p = 0.052$	256 (17.50)
LVEF < 40%	1 (4.50) $p = 0.003$	2 (16.70) $p < 0.001$	3 (9.10) $p < 0.001$	555 (37.80)
Renal failure (any)	3 (13.60) $p = 0.316$	1 (8.30) $p = 0.127$	4 (12.10) $p = 0.127$	371 (25.30)
Charlson comorbidity index [points]	2.55 ± 2.41 $p < 0.001$	3.67 ± 3.53 $p = 0.013$	3.03 ± 2.85 $p < 0.001$	5.14 ± 3.76
		TLE Indications		
CIED-related infection (any)	4 (18.20) $p = 0.917$	2 (16.70) $p = 0.964$	6 (18.20) $p = 0.817$	314 (21.40)
Non-infectious indications	18 (81.80) $p = 0.917$	10 (83.30) $p = 0.964$	27 (81.80) $p = 0.817$	1153 (78.60)
		System		
Pacemaker-with RA lead	18 (81.80) $p = 0.028$	8 (66.70) $p = 0.621$	26 (78.80) $p = 0.012$	812 (55.40)
Pacemaker-without RA lead and only abandoned PM lead	2 (9.10) $p = 0.974$	3 (25.00) $p = 0.294$	4 (12.10) $p = 0.663$	164 (11.20)
ICD-with RA lead	0 (0.00) $p = 0.170$	0 (0.00) $p = 0.424$	1 (3.00) $p = 0.210$	170 (11.60)
ICD-without RA lead and only HV lead	1 (4.50) $p = 0.409$	1 (8.30) $p = 0.982$	1 (3.00) $p = 0.379$	187 (12.70)
ICD-CRT-D pacing system	1 (4.50) $p = 0.726$	0 (0.00) $p = 0.562$	1 (3.00) $p = 0.377$	132 (9.90)
Number of leads in the heart before TLE	2.14 ± 0.94 $p = 0.690$	2.08 ± 0.67 $p = 0.684$	2.15 ± 0.83 $p = 0.365$	1.92 ± 0.69
Abandoned leads before TLE	5 (22.70) $p = 0.019$	4 (33.30) $p = 0.004$	9 (27.30) $p < 0.001$	106 (7.20)
Large lead loop on X-rays before TLE	3 (13.60) $p = 0.015$	1 (8.30) $p = 0.754$	4 (12.10) $p < 0.001$	39 (2.70)
Small lead loop on X-rays before TLE	5 (22.70) $p = 0.250$	1 (8.30) $p = 0.978$	6 (18.20) $p = 0.452$	180 (12.30)
Number of procedures before lead extraction	3.00 ± 2.00 $p < 0.001$	2.83 ± 1.34 $p = 0.003$	2.90 ± 1.77 $p < 0.001$	1.79 ± 0.91
Dwell time of the oldest lead per patient before TLE [months]	214.9 ± 91.86 $p < 0.001$	217.9 ± 106.2 $p < 0.001$	215.0 ± 96.87 $p < 0.001$	109.8 ± 76.15
Mean implant duration (per patient) before TLE [months]	201.25 ± 81.14 $p < 0.001$	178.0 ± 62.89 $p < 0.001$	191.4 ± 75.59 $p < 0.001$	103.3 ± 68.79
Global implant duration (sum of lead dwell times) [years]	36.96 ± 23.12 $p < 0.001$	30.56 ± 13.85 $p < 0.001$	35.12 ± 20.50 $p < 0.001$	16.60 ± 13.29

Abbreviations: CIED—cardiac implantable electronic device, CRT—cardiac resynchronization therapy, ICD—implantable cardioverter-defibrillator, LVEF—left ventricular ejection fraction, NYHA—New York Heart Association class, PM—pacemaker, RA—right atrium, TLE—transvenous lead extraction.

Table 2. Patient/system/history of pacing.

	Hemorrhagic Complication (Cardiac/Vascular Wall Tear)	Tricuspid Valve Damage	All Major Complications (Mixed Damages 1 Case)	Control Group (No Major Complications)
	A N = 22 Mean ± SD n (%)	B N = 12 Mean ± SD n (%)	C N = 33 Mean ± SD n (%)	D N = 1467 Mean ± SD n (%)
	TLE Procedure Potential Risk Factors of Major TLE Complications and Procedure Complicity			
Number of leads extracted per patient	2.30 ± 1.58 $p = 0.079$	2.39 ± 1.81 $p = 0.189$	2.21 ± 1.34 $p = 0.008$	1.63 ± 0.71
Three or more leads extracted	5 (22.79) $p = 0.091$	2 (16.70) $p = 0.739$	7 (21.20) $p = 0.056$	141 (9.60)
Extraction of leads with redundant loop (large)	3 (13.60) $p = 0.083$	1 (8.30) $p = 0.696$	4 (12.10) $p = 0.004$	35 (2.40)
Extraction of abandoned lead(s) (any)	4 (18.20) $p = 0.094$	4 (33.30) $p = 0.002$	8 (24.20) $p < 0.001$	99 (6.70)
HV therapy (ICD) lead extracted	2 (9.10) $p = 0.043$	1 (8.30) $p = 0.158$	3 (9.10) $p = 0.010$	462 (31.50)

Table 2. Cont.

	Hemorrhagic Complication (Cardiac/Vascular Wall Tear)	Tricuspid Valve Damage	All Major Complications (Mixed Damages 1 Case)	Control Group (No Major Complications)
Atrial lead extracted (any)	19 (86.40) $p = 0.018$	6 (50.00) $p = 0.080$	25 (75.80) $p = 0.044$	867 (59.10)
CS (LV pacing) lead extracted	1 (4.50) $p = 0.964$	0 (0.00) $p = 0.737$	1 (3.00) $p = 0.640$	97 (6.60)
Dwell time of the oldest lead extracted	214.9 (91.86) $p < 0.001$	217.9 ± 106.2 $p = 0.001$	215.0 ± 96.87 $p = 0 < 001$	108.8 ± 75.74
Average (per patient) dwell time of lead extracted	201.3 (81.14) $p < 0.001$	176.9 ± 63.75 $p = 0.001$	191.0 ± 75.91 $p < 0.001$	103.8 ± 69.47
Cumulative dwell time of lead extracted (in years)	36.34 (23.81) $p < 0.001$	28.72 ± 14.88 $p = 0.001$	34.05 ± 21.37 $p < 0.001$	14.96 ± 13.23
SAFeTY TLE calculator of risk of MC of TLE—[number of points]	13.03 (4.73) $p < 0.001$	11.42 ± 4.60 $p = 0.001$	12.31 ± 4.69 $p < 0.001$	6.11 ± 4.32
Risk of MC calculated by SAFeTY TLE calculator (%)	9.40 (12.70) $p < 0.001$	6.17 ± 6.06 $p < 0.001$	8.06 ± 10.89 $p < 0.001$	1.79 ± 2.58
Analysis of Extracted Leads: Lead Model, Tip Location and Mechanism of Tip Fixation.				
Tip Location				
RAA	22 (47.73) $p = 0.139$	7 (30.43) $p = 0.355$	29 (42.64) $p = 0.355$	901 (37.04)
BB	1 (2.27) $p = 0.693$	0 (0.00) $p = 0.911$	1 (1.47) $p = 0.911$	15 (0.62)
CS	1 (2.27) $p = 0.967$	0 (0.00) $p = 0.811$	1 (1.47) $p = 0.811$	25 (1.03)
CSO	1 (2.27) $p = 0.772$	0 (.00) $p = 0.783$	1 (1.47) $p = 0.783$	44 (1.82)
RVA	17 (38.64) $p = 0.505$	10 (43.48) $p = 480$	27 (39.71) $p = 0.483$	1069 (43.69)
Outside RVA	2 (4.55) $p = 0.231$	6 (26.09) $p = 0.985$	8 (11.76) $p = 0.985$	274 (11.31)
LV vein	1 (2.27 $p = 0.726$	0 (0.00) $p = 0.390$	1 (1.47) $p = 0.390$	108 (4.46)
Lead Type				
BP pacemaker leads	39 (86.67) $p = 0.106$	18 (78.26) $p = 0.146$	57 (83.82) $p = 0.146$	1828 (75.04)
VDD pacemaker leads	0 (0.00) $p = 0.952$	0 (0.00) $p = 0.730$	0 (0.00) $p = 0.730$	30 (1.19)
UP pacemaker leads	4 (8.89) $p = 0.256$	4 (17.39) $p = 0.007$	8 (11.76) $p = 0.007$	104 (4.19)
ICD leads single coil	2 (4.44) $p = 0.231$	0 (0.00) $p = 0.053$	2 (2.94) $p = 0.053$	274 (11.25)
ICD leads dual coil	0 (0.00) $p = 0.084$	1 (4.35) $p = 0.077$	1 (1.47) $p = 0.077$	200 (8.21)
All	45 (100)	23 (100.0)	68 (100.0)	2436 (100.0)
Tip Fixation Mode				
Active fixation lead	9 (20.00) $p < 0.001$	11 (47.83) $p < 0.001$	20 (29.41) $p < 0.001$	1408 (57.73)
Passive fixation lead	36 (80.00) $p \leq 0.001$	12 (52.17) $p < 0.001$	48 (70.59) $p < 0.001$	1028 (42.18)

Abbreviations: BB—Bachman Bundle, BP—bipolar, CS—coronary sinus, CSO—coronary sinus ostium, ICD—implantable cardioverter-defibrillator, LV vein—cardiac vein located on LV wall utilized for LV pacing PM—pacemaker, RA—right atrium, RAA-right atrial appendage, RVA—RV apex, UP—unipolar, VDD—single-lead atrial triggered ventricular pacing, TLE—transvenous lead extraction.

Our analysis of the effectiveness and TLE-related complications demonstrated that procedure duration (skin-to-skin time, sheath-to-sheath time) and mean extraction time per lead were much longer in patients with the two types of major complications. The occurrence of any technical problem during TLE, lead-to-lead binding (intraoperative diagnosis), fracture of the extracted lead, three or more technical problems, the need to use Evolution or TightRail or lasso catheters/snares were dramatically more frequent in groups with CVWT or TVD. It seems to be related to lead implant duration, proliferation of tissue scar around the lead and necessity to use slightly more aggressive tools. Byrd dilator torsion/collapse is more frequent if ventricular leads are extracted, which is easy to explain by the anatomy (bend) and extracted lead route (Table 4).

Table 3. TTE and TEE before TLE.

	Hemorrhagic Complication (Cardiac/Vascular Wall Tear)	Tricuspid Valve Damage	All Major Complications (Mixed Damages 1 Case)	Control Group (No Major Complications)
Groups of patients	A N = 22 Mean ± SD n (%)	B N = 12 Mean ± SD n (%)	C N = 33 Mean ± SD n (%)	D N = 1467 Mean ± SD n (%)
TTE before TLE				
LVEF average [%]	59.43 ± 10.85 $p = 0.002$	56.00 ± 11.78 $p = 0.049$	58.06 ± 11.29 $p < 0.001$	49.07 ± 15.96
TVR-mild (0,1)	15 (68.20) $p = 0.214$	8 (66.70) $p = 0.214$	22 (66.70) $p = 0.153$	771 (52.60)
TVR-intermediate/mid (2,3)	6 (27.30) $p = 0.417$	4 (33.30) $p = 0.469$	10 (30.30) 0.469	558 (38.00)
TVR-severe (4)	0 (0.00) $p = 0.382$	0 (0.00) $p = 0.215$	0 (0.00) $p = 0.215$	104 (7.10)
Lack of examination	1 (4.50) $p = 0.610$	0 (0.00) $p = 0.997$	1 (3.00) $p = 0.997$	67 (4.60)
RVSP [mm Hg]	27.24 ± 8.57 $p = 0.075$	26.08 (7.12) $p = 0.010$	27.06 ± 7.98 $p = 0.010$	32.07 (11.82)
TEE Findings before TLE				
Oscillating tissue scar on the lead	7 (38.80) $p = 0.080$	3 (25.00) $p = 0.044$	10 (30.30) $p < 0.044$	231 (15.70)
Lead thickening (encapsulation)	14 (63.60) $p < 0.001$	9 (75.00) $p < 0.001$	22 (66.70) $p < 0.001$	398 (27.10)
Lead-to-lead binding	10 (45.50) $p < 0.001$	5 (41.70) $p < 0.001$	15 (45.50) $p < 0.001$	208 (14.20)
Lead adhering to any heart structure	11 (50.00) $p < 0.001$	10 (83.30) $p < 0.001$	20 (60.60) $p < 0.001$	242 (16.50)
Lead adhering to tricuspid valve	5 (22.70) $p = 0.031$	6 (50.00) $p < 0.001$	11 (33.30) $p < 0.001$	115 (7.80)
Lead adhering to superior vena cava	5 (22.70) $p = 0.004$	4 (33.30) $p < 0.001$	9 (27.30) $p < 0.001$	83 (5.70)
Lead adhering to RA wall	9 (40.90) $p < 0.001$	1 (8.30) $p < 0.001$	10 (30.30) $p < 0.001$	92 (6.30)
Lead adhering to RV wall	7 (31.80) $p = 0.002$	8 (66.70) $p < 0.001$	14 (42.40) $p < 0.001$	140 (9.50)
Tissue scar occurrence (any form) (possible multiple options)	3.272 ± 1.725 $p < 0.001$	3.917 ± 1.647 $p < 0.001$	3.515 ± 1.587 $p < 0.001$	1.188 ± 1.225
Occurrence of any form of tissue scar	14 (63.60) $p = 0.026$	10 (83.30) $p < 0.001$	23 (69.70) $p < 0.001$	558 (38.00)
Perforation of RV wall/ECHO finding	1 (4.50) $p = 0.578$	1 (8.30) $p = 0.591$	2 (6.10) $p = 0.591$	154 (10.50)

Abbreviations: LVEF—left ventricular ejection fraction, RA—right atrium, RV—right ventricle, RVSP—right ventricular systolic pressure, TVR—tricuspid valve regurgitation.

TEE and blood pressure monitoring during TLE showed that pulling on the right atrial appendage (RAA), TV and RV wall as well as pulling on the other lead were more common in patients with CVWT and TVD. A transient drop in blood pressure during TLE is usually caused by pulling on the RV wall, rarely on the SVC with a significant reduction of its diameter or by any reflex action (Spearman rank correlation coefficient r = 0.320; $p < 0.001$). This was confirmed by the drop in blood pressure in TVD group vs. control group. However, a decrease in blood pressure can be a warming sign of bleeding into the pericardial sac, right pleura or mediastinum. The drop in blood pressure was significantly higher in patients with CVWT because of blood loss (Table 4).

Table 4. TLE procedure complexity, efficacy, complications and mortality for any reason.

Groups of patients	Hemorrhagic Complication (Cardiac/Vascular Wall Tear) A N = 22 Mean ± SD n (%)	Tricuspid Valve Damage B N = 12 Mean ± SD n (%)	All Major Complications (Mixed Damages 1 Case) C N = 33 Mean ± SD n (%)	Control Group (No Major Complications) D N = 1467 Mean ± SD n (%)
TLE Procedure Complexity and Efficacy				
Procedure duration (skin-to-skin)	104.4 ± 52.24 $p < 0.001$	81.33 ± 31.76 $p = 0.004$	94.61 ± 46.62 $p < 0.001$	60.93 ± 25.93
Procedure duration (sheath-to-sheath)	55.53 ± 55.93 $p < 0.001$	29.92 ± 21.16 $p < 0.001$	46.67 ± 48.69 $p < 0.001$	13.91 ± 21.32
Average time of single lead extr. (sheath-to-sheath/number of extracted leads)	25.62 ± 21.63 $p < 0.001$	16.69 ± 13.00 $p < 0.001$	21.79 ± 19.19 $p < 0.001$	8.40 ± 13.26
Technical problem during TLE (any)	14 (63.60) $p < 0.001$	8 (66.70) $p < 0.001$	21 (63.60) $p < 0.001$	321 (21.90)
Lead-to-lead binding (intraoperative diagnosis)	11 (50.00) $p < 0.001$	5 (41.70) $p < 0.001$	16 (48.50) $p < 0.001$	106 (7.20)
Block at venous entry site	4 (18.20) $p = 0.497$	3 (25.00) $p = 0.497$	7 (21.20) $p = 0.134$	165 (11.20)
Fracture of extracted lead	7 (31.80) $p < 0.001$	3 (25.00) $p < 0.001$	10 (30.30) $p < 0.001$	65 (4.40)
Byrd dilator torsion/collapse	2 (9.10) $p = 0.544$	4 (33.30) $p = 0.544$	6 (18.20) $p = 0.544$	61 (4.20)
Three or more technical problems	3 (13.60) $p < 0.001$	1 (8.30) $p < 0.001$	4 (12.10) $p < 0.001$	25 (1.70)
Use of Evolution (old and new) or TightRail	3 (13.60) $p = 0.007$	3 (25.00) $p = 0.007$	5 (15.20) $p = 0.003$	34 (2.30)
Use of lasso catheters/snares	5 (22.70) $p < 0.001$	3 (25.00) $p < 0.001$	8 (24.20) $p < 0.001$	47 (3.20)
Temporary pacing during procedure	3 (13.60) 0.348	5 (41.70) $p = 0.348$	8 (24.20) $p = 0.3876$	361 (24.60)
TEE and Blood Pressure Monitoring				
RAA pulling/drawing	15 (5) $p < 0.001$	3 (25.00) $p < 0.001$	18 (54.50) $p = 0.012$	472 (32.20)
TV pulling/drawing	6 (27.30) $p < 0.001$	11 (91.70) $p < 0.001$	16 (48.50) $p < 0.001$	100 (6.80)
RV wall pulling	10 (45.50) $p = 0.015$	8 (66.70) $p = 0.015$	17 (51.50) $p < 0.001$	317 (21.60)
Other lead pulling	10 (45.50)	5 (41.70) $p < 0.001$	15 (45.50) $p < 0.001$	116 (7.90)
Pulling/drawing of heart structures or other lead (possible multiple options)	1.864 ± 1.46 $p < 0.001$	2.250 ± 1.224 $p < 0.001$	2.00 ± 1.350 $p < 0.001$	0.670 ± 0.928
Max blood pressure drop during TLE [mm Hg]	54.43 ± 23.42 $p < 0.001$	38.89 ± 21.03 $p < 0.001$	48.38 ± 22.64 $p < 0.001$	20.79 ± 14.53
Significant blood pressure drop during TLE (different reasons)	13 (59.10) $p < 0.001$	3 (25.00) $p < 0.001$	15 (45.50) $p < 0.001$	137 (9.30)
TLE Efficacy and Complications				
Worsening TR for 1 degree	2 (9.10) $p = 0.956$	0 (0.00) $p = 0.956$	2 (6.10) $p = 0.908$	104 (7.10)
Worsening TR for 2 degrees	0 (0.00) $p = 0.95$	4 (33.30) $p = 0.95$	4 (12.10) $p = 0.002$	31 (2.10)
Worsening TR for 3 degrees	1 (4.50) $p < 0.001$	8 (66.70) $p < 0.001$	8 (24.20) $p < 0.001$	0 (0.00)
Tricuspid valve damage during TLE (severe)	0 (0.00) N	12 (100.0) $p < 0.001$	12 (36.40) $p < 0.001$	0 (0.00)
Procedure-related death (intra-, post-procedural)	0 (0.00) N	0 (0.00) N	0 (0.00) N	0 (0.00)
Clinical success	21 (95.50) $p = 0.114$	0 (0.00) $p = 0.114$	21 (63.60) $p < 0.001$	1463 (99.70)
Complete procedural success	20 (90.90) $p = 0.322$	0 (0.00) $p = 0.322$	20 (60.60) $p < 0.001$	1422 (96.90)
Short-, Mid-and Long-Term Mortality after TLE (Any Reason)				
First day (first 48 h)	0 (0.00) $p = 0862$	0 (0.00) $p = 0.862$	0 (0.00) $p = 0.832$	2 (0.14)
Mortality at 1 month after TLE (2–30 days)	0 (0.00) $p = 0.78$	0 (0.00) $p = 0.780$	0 (0.00) $p = 0.993$	23 (1.57)
Mortality at 1 year after TLE (31–365 days)	1 (4.55) 0.985	1 (8.33) 0.985	2 (6.06) 0.845	99 (6.75)
Mortality at 3 years TLE (366–1095 days)	1 (4.55) 0.855	0 (0.00) $p = 0.855$	1 (3.03) $p = 0.841$	116 (7.91)
Mortality > 3 years after TLE (> 1095 days)	0 (0.00) 0.673	1 (8.33) $p = 0.673$	1 (3.03) $p = 0.888$	60 (4.09)

Abbreviations: RAA—right atrial appendage, RV—right ventricle, TLE—transvenous lead extraction, TR—tricuspid regurgitation, TV—tricuspid valve.

Assessment of TV function during and after TLE revealed that the worsening of tricuspid valve regurgitation (TVR) by one degree was similar in all study subgroups. TVD after TLE was considered as major complication if TR deteriorated by at least two degrees to grade 4.

Irrespective of the organizational model of TLE procedures and despite the occurrence of severe major complications, there were no procedure-related deaths. Effective surgical management of CVWT resulted in the rates of clinical and procedural success comparable to those in the control group.

An analysis of short-, mid-and long-term mortality (for any reason) after TLE demonstrated that there were no deaths within 30 days. Mid-and long-term mortality in patients with major complications was similar to that in the control group (Table 4).

A summary of the most important risk factors for TLE complications is presented schematically in Figure 1.

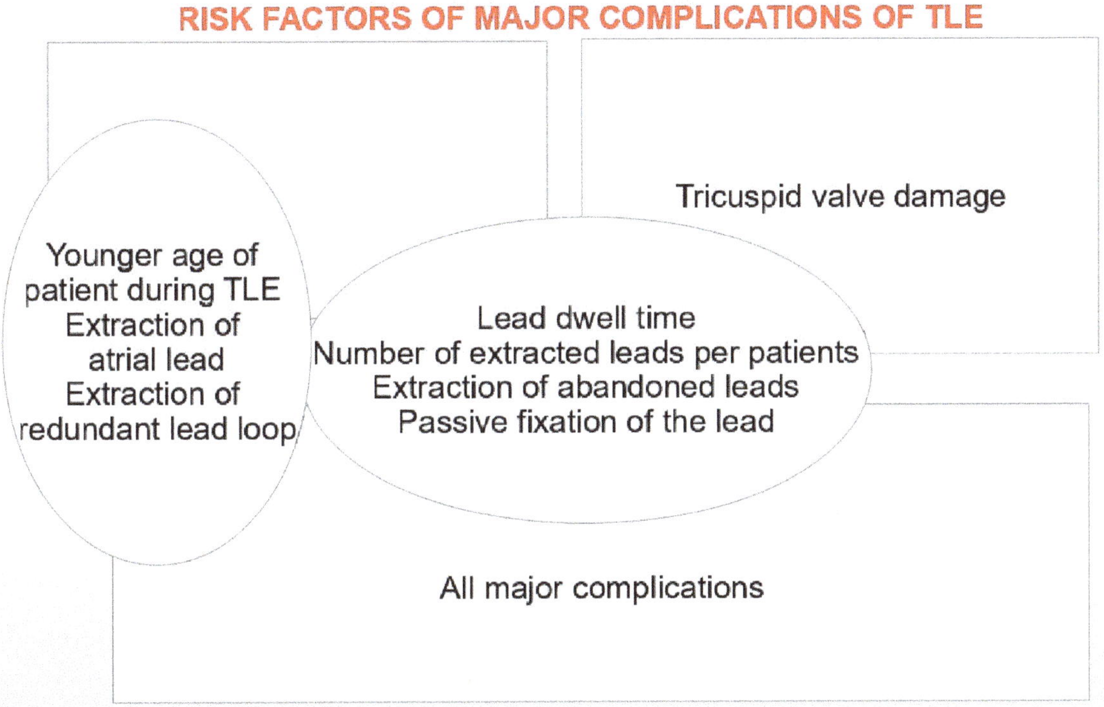

RISK FACTORS OF MAJOR COMPLICATIONS OF TLE

Tricuspid valve damage

**Younger age of patient during TLE
Extraction of atrial lead
Extraction of redundant lead loop**

**Lead dwell time
Number of extracted leads per patients
Extraction of abandoned leads
Passive fixation of the lead**

All major complications

Figure 1. Graphical presentation of the main results

4. Discussion

Transvenous lead extraction is an integral part of the management of CIED-related problems [1–5]. Cardiac and venous injuries during lead extraction are complications with potentially serious consequences. So far, there has been no comprehensive analysis of TLE complications that would include TLE-related TV damage apart from injuries to the SVC/other vessels. Not much is known about risk factors for TLE-related TV damage [12–18].

This study showed that patients with hemorrhagic complications were significantly younger and received their first CIED earlier than in the control group. There were twice as many women as men, among them significantly fewer patients with low LVEF and class NYHA class III or IV, and they were more likely to have procedural risk factors (abandoned leads, excessive loops of the leads, more previous CIED-related procedures). The younger age of the patient during TLE is one of the risk factors, especially for CVWT, because in young people, more intense proliferation of connective tissue is observed, with more adhesion of the lead to the walls of the heart and vessels. This factor, as well as lead dwell time and female gender, was included in the previously constructed risk scale of major complications SAFeTY-TLE [23].

Patients with worsening TVR were older but received their CIED nine years earlier than the control group. In many ways, patients with TVD are somewhere between those with CVWT and the control group. The number of leads extracted per patient, need to extract three or more leads, extraction of leads with redundant loops, extraction of abandoned lead(s) and extraction of atrial leads were intraprocedural risk factors for CVWT and TVD; however, extended implant duration was the strongest predictor of both CVWT and TVD. Extraction of RAA leads, bipolar (BP) or unipolar (UP), and passive fixation leads indicated the risk of CVWT (the most frequent finding was RAA tear). Right ventricular lead tips placed in a different position than the apex, passive fixation and UP leads were the predictors TVD.

In the two groups with major complications the state of the tricuspid valve at baseline was comparable, LVEF was higher and right ventricular systolic pressure was lower. Moreover, patients with CVWT or TVD were significantly more likely to have any form of tissue scar (oscillating tissue scar on the lead, lead thickening, lead-to-lead binding and lead adherence to any heart structure). Procedure duration was much longer in patients with the two types of major complications. The occurrence of any technical problem during TLE, lead-to-lead binding (intraoperative diagnosis), fracture of extracted leads, three or more technical problems, need to use Evolution (old and new) or TightRail or lasso catheters/snares were dramatically more frequent in patients with CVWT or TVD. A frequent technical problem during complicated TLEs was lead breakage. This is probably related to similar risk factors, as shown in the literature [32].

Pulling on the RAA, TV and RV wall as well as other lead was more common in patients with CVWT and TVD. A transient drop in blood pressure during TLE is usually caused by pulling on the RV wall, rarely on the SVC with a significant reduction of its diameter or by any reflex action. The BP drop was significantly higher in patients with CVWD because of blood loss.

According to recent reports, the use of a laser is associated with high efficiency also in the removal of leads with a long dwell time, although the rate of major complications remains relatively high (3.3%) [33]. If excimer laser energy is not applied, major complications other than tear of the SVC and anonymous vein seem to be more common [21–27]. The available guidelines and medical literature focus on cardiac/vascular wall tear but not on worsening TR after TLE [1–5,7–11]. On the other hand, several reports (experience with 100–200 TLE procedures) have described a wide spectrum of TLE-related TVD (Givon—15% [14], Park—11.5% [12], Franceschi—9.1% [18], Rodriguez—6% [17], Coffey—5.6% [16], Pecha—1.9% [13], Regoli—1.2% [15]), but there has been little discussion about risk factors for TLE-related TVD. In the 2018 EHRA expert consensus statement on lead extraction—recommendations on definitions, endpoints, research trial design, and data collection requirements for clinical scientific studies and registries: endorsed by APHRS/HRS/LAHRS [5]—we find much lower percentages: flail tricuspid valve leaflet requiring intervention: 0.03% (being major complication) and worsening tricuspid valve function: 0.02–0.59 % (being minor complication).

There are two large studies of the occurrence and management of cardiac/vascular wall damage (CVWD) during lead extraction using mainly laser technique [7,9]. Brunner et al. reported a 0.8% incidence rate of complications requiring rescue intervention (mean implant duration time 4.9 years). SVC laceration was most frequent (80%), whereas RA and RV wall damage was rare [7]. Bashir et al. reported CVWD in 3% of TLE patients, but mean implant duration time was much longer than in the previous study (10.8 years). Overall, 84.8% of devastating injuries were cardiac tamponade [9].

Damage to the tricuspid valve during extraction is estimated to range from 3.5% to 15%, and even to 19% [4,5,12–18]. In this study, we noted worsening TR by 1 degree (7.29%), by 2 degrees (2.50%), by 3 degrees (0.61%) and severe TVD fulfilling the criteria of TV repair (0.82%), which is less than previously reported [4,5,12–18]. The need for surgical intervention in such cases is rare [12–18,34].

This study and literature review [12–18,34] indicate that one of most important safety challenges during lead removal is still the unsolved problem of TLE-related TV damage which is caused by fibrous adhesion of the lead to the TV leaflet. Excessive pulling on the lead may cause leaflet disruption, and wrapping of the leaflet around the dilating sheath during rotational lead extraction will do the same. Excellent teamwork combined with TEE monitoring may help warn the extractor about potentially harmful situations leading to TV damage [28–31]. The lead to be removed can be fused to the chordae tendinae or even to the head of the papillary muscle and damages to these structures may go unnoticed. According to recent report, monitoring of TLE by intracardiac echocardiography may even more precisely visualize the growth of he leads to the walls of the heart, including the tricuspid valve [35].

5. Conclusions

The risk factors for cardiac/vascular wall tear and tricuspid valve damage during TLE are similar and include extended implant duration and other procedural and system-dependent factors: number of extracted leads, extraction of leads with redundant loops, extraction of abandoned lead (s), extraction of atrial leads. The immediate cause of major complications is increased proliferation of the connective tissue resulting from the long presence of the leads in the heart and making them grow into the heart structures. Nevertheless, TVD patients are similarly old as the control group—proliferation of tissue scar surrounding the lead is similar to that observed in much younger patients with CVWD.

Both TVD and CVWT occur more frequently during extraction of pacemaker passive (and unipolar) fixation leads. ICD lead extraction does not generate higher risk of TVD or CVWT. The occurrence of TLE complications does not affect the long-term survival of patients.

6. Study Limitations

The database of the study group was integrated prospectively, but analysis was performed retrospectively. The main limitation is the lack of echocardiographic follow-up with late reassessment of TVD.

Author Contributions: Ł.T.—writing-original draft preparation; A.P.—investigation; W.J.—methodology, statistical study; D.N.—data curation, K.T.—data curation; P.S.—data curation; J.K.—investigation; K.D.—investigation; M.P.—data curation; A.K.—writing-review and editing. All authors have read and agreed to the published version of the manuscript.

Funding: This research received no external funding.

Institutional Review Board Statement: The study was conducted according to the guidelines of the Declaration of Helsinki, and approved by the of Bioethics Committee at the Regional Medical Chamber in Lublin protocol number 288/2018/KB/VII.

Informed Consent Statement: Informed consent was obtained from all subjects involved in the study.

Data Availability Statement: Readers can access the data supporting the conclusions of the study at www.usuwanieelektrod.pl.

Conflicts of Interest: The authors declare no conflict of interest.

References

1. Love, C.J.; Wilkoff, B.L.; Byrd, C.L.; Belott, P.H.; Brinker, J.A.; Fearnot, N.E.; Friedman, R.A.; Furman, S.; Goode, L.B.; Hayes, D.L.; et al. Recommendations for extraction of chronically implanted transvenous pacing and defibrillator leads: Indications, facilities, training. North American Society of Pacing and Electrophysiology Lead Extraction Conference Faculty. *Pacing Clin. Electrophysiol.* **2000**, *23*, 544–551.
2. Wilkoff, B.L.; Love, C.J.; Byrd, C.L.; Bongiorni, M.G.; Carrillo, R.G.; Crossley, G.H., 3rd; Epstein, L.M.; Friedman, R.A.; Kennergren, C.E.; Mitkowski, P.; et al. Heart Rhythm Society; American Heart Association. Transvenous lead extraction: Heart Rhythm Society expert consensus on facilities, training, indications, and patient management: This document was endorsed by the American Heart Association (AHA). *Heart Rhythm* **2009**, *6*, 1085–1104. [CrossRef]
3. Deharo, J.C.; Bongiorni, M.G.; Rozkovec, A.; Bracke, F.; Defaye, P.; Fernandez-Lozano, I.; Golzio, P.G.; Hansky, B.; Kennergren, C.; Manolis, A.S.; et al. European Heart Rhythm Association. Pathways for training and accreditation for transvenous lead extraction: A European Heart Rhythm Association position paper. *Europace* **2012**, *14*, 124–134. [PubMed]
4. Kusumoto, F.M.; Schoenfeld, M.H.; Wilkoff, B.; Berul, C.I.; Birgersdotter-Green, U.M.; Carrillo, R.; Cha, Y.M.; Clancy, J.; Deharo, J.C.; Ellenbogen, K.A.; et al. 2017 HRS expert consensus statement on cardiovascular implantable electronic device lead management and extraction. *Heart Rhythm* **2017**, *14*, e503–e551. [CrossRef]
5. Bongiorni, M.G.; Burri, H.; Deharo, J.C.; Starck, C.; Kennergren, C.; Saghy, L.; Rao, A.; Tascini, C.; Lever, N.; Kutarski, A.; et al. 2018 EHRA expert consensus statement on lead extraction: Recommendations on definitions, endpoints, research trial design, and data collection requirements for clinical scientific studies and registries: Endorsed by APHRS/HRS/LAHRS. *Europace* **2012**, *14*, 994–1001. [CrossRef]
6. Nowosielecka, D.; Polewczyk, A.; Jacheć, W.; Tułecki, Ł.; Kleinrok, A.; Kutarski, A. Echocardiographic findings in patients with cardiac implantable electronic devices-analysis of factors predisposing to lead-associated changes. *Clin. Physiol. Funct. Imaging* **2021**, *41*, 25–41. [CrossRef] [PubMed]
7. Brunner, M.P.; Cronin, E.M.; Wazni, O.; Baranowski, B.; Saliba, W.I.; Sabik, J.F.; Lindsay, B.D.; Wilkoff, B.L.; Tarakji, K.G. Outcomes of patients requiring emergent surgical or endovascular intervention for catastrophic complications during transvenous lead extraction. *Heart Rhythm* **2014**, *11*, 419–425. [CrossRef]
8. Wang, W.; Wang, X.; Modry, D.; Wang, S. Cardiopulmonary bypass standby avoids fatality due to vascular laceration in laser-assisted lead extraction. *J. Card. Surg.* **2014**, *29*, 274–278. [CrossRef]
9. Bashir, J.; Fedoruk, L.M.; Ofiesh, J.; Karim, S.S.; Tyers, G.F.O. Classification and surgical repair of injuries sustained during transvenous lead extraction. *Circ. Arrhythmia Electrophysiol.* **2016**, *9*, e003741. [CrossRef] [PubMed]
10. Hosseini, S.M.; Rozen, G.; Kaadan, M.I.; Galvin, J.; Ruskin, J.N. Safety and In-Hospital Outcomes of Transvenous Lead Extraction for Cardiac Implantable Device-Related Infections: Analysis of 13 Years of Inpatient Data in the United States. *JACC Clin. Electrophysiol.* **2019**, *5*, 1450–1458. [CrossRef]
11. Hauser, R.G.; Katsiyiannis, W.T.; Gornick, C.C.; Almquist, A.K.; Kallinen, L.M. Deaths and cardiovascular injuries due to device assisted implantable cardioverter–defibrillator and pacemaker lead extraction. *Europace* **2010**, *12*, 395–401. [CrossRef] [PubMed]
12. Park, S.J.; Gentry, J.L., 3rd; Varma, N.; Wazni, O.; Tarakji, K.G.; Mehta, A.; Mick, S.; Grimm, R.; Wilkoff, B.L. Transvenous Extraction of Pacemaker and Defibrillator Leads and the Risk of Tricuspid Valve Regurgitation. *JACC Clin. Electrophysiol.* **2018**, *4*, 1421–1428. [CrossRef]
13. Pecha, S.; Castro, L.; Gosau, N.; Linder, M.; Vogler, J.; Willems, S.; Reichenspurner, H.; Hakmi, S. Evaluation of tricuspid valve regurgitation following laser lead extraction†. *Eur. J. Cardiothorac. Surg.* **2017**, *51*, 1108–1111. [CrossRef]
14. Givon, A.; Vedernikova, N.; Luria, D.; Vatury, O.; Kuperstein, R.; Feinberg, M.S.; Eldar, M.; Glikson, M.; Nof, E. Tricuspid Regurgitation following Lead Extraction: Risk Factors and Clinical Course. *Isr. Med. Assoc. J.* **2016**, *18*, 18–22. [PubMed]
15. Regoli, F.; Caputo, M.; Conte, G.; Faletra, F.F.; Moccetti, T.; Pasotti, E.; Cassina, T.; Casso, G.; Schlotterbeck, H.; Engeler, A.; et al. Clinical utility of routine use of continuous transesophageal echocardiography monitoring during transvenous lead extraction procedure. *Heart Rhythm* **2015**, *12*, 313–320. [CrossRef]
16. Coffey, J.O.; Sager, S.J.; Gangireddy, S.; Levine, A.; Viles-Gonzalez, J.F.; Fischer, A. The impact of transvenous lead extraction on tricuspid valve function. *Pacing Clin. Electrophysiol.* **2014**, *37*, 19–24. [CrossRef]
17. Rodriguez, Y.; Mesa, J.; Arguelles, E.; Carrillo, R.G. Tricuspid insufficiency after laser lead extraction. *Pacing Clin. Electrophysiol.* **2013**, *36*, 939–944. [CrossRef]
18. Franceschi, F.; Thuny, F.; Giorgi, R.; Sanaa, I.; Peyrouse, E.; Assouan, X.; Prévôt, S.; Bastard, E.; Habib, G.; Deharo, J.C. Incidence, risk factors and outcome of traumatic tricuspid regurgitation after percutaneous ventricular lead removal. *J. Am. Coll. Cardiol.* **2009**, *53*, 2168–2174. [CrossRef]
19. Zucchelli, G.; Di Cori, A.; Segreti, L.; Laroche, C.; Blomstrom-Lundqvist, C.; Kutarski, A.; Regoli, F.; Butter, C.; Defaye, P.; Pasquié, J.L.; et al. ELECTRa Investigators. Major cardiac and vascular complications after transvenous lead extraction: Acute outcome and predictive factors from the ESC-EHRA ELECTRa (European Lead Extraction ConTRolled) registry. *Europace* **2019**, *21*, 771–780. [CrossRef]
20. Jacheć, W.; Polewczyk, A.; Polewczyk, M.; Tomasik, A.; Janion, M.; Kutarski, A. Risk Factors Predicting Complications of Transvenous Lead Extraction. *Biomed Res. Int.* **2018**, *2018*, 8796704. [CrossRef] [PubMed]

21. Brunner, M.P.; Cronin, E.M.; Duarte, V.E.; Yu, C.; Tarakji, K.G.; Martin, D.O.; Callahan, T.; Cantillon, D.J.; Niebauer, M.J.; Saliba, W.I.; et al. Clinical predictors of adverse patient outcomes in an experience of more than 5000 chronic endovascular pacemaker and defibrillator lead extractions. *Heart Rhythm* **2014**, *11*, 799–805. [CrossRef]
22. Wazni, O.; Epstein, L.M.; Carrillo, R.G.; Love, C.; Adler, S.W.; Riggio, D.W.; Karim, S.S.; Bashir, J.; Greenspon, A.J.; DiMarco, J.P.; et al. Lead extraction in the contemporary setting: The LExICon study: An observational retrospective study of consecutive laser lead extractions. *J. Am. Coll. Cardiol.* **2010**, *55*, 579–586. [CrossRef]
23. Jacheć, W.; Polewczyk, A.; Polewczyk, M.; Tomasik, A.; Kutarski, A. Transvenous Lead Extraction, S.A.FeTY Score for Risk Stratification and Proper Patient Selection for Removal Procedures Using Mechanical Tools. *J. Clin. Med.* **2020**, *9*, 361. [CrossRef] [PubMed]
24. Sidhu, B.S.; Ayis, S.; Gould, J.; Elliott, M.K.; Mehta, V.; Kennergren, C.; Butter, C.; Deharo, J.C.; Kutarski, A.; Maggioni, A.P.; et al. ELECTRa Investigators Group. Risk stratification of patients undergoing transvenous lead extraction with the ELECTRa Registry Outcome Score (EROS): An ESC EHRA EORP European lead extraction ConTRolled, E.L.ECTRa registry analysis. *Europace* **2021**, euab037, online ahead of print. [CrossRef]
25. Kancharla, K.; Acker, N.G.; Li, Z.; Samineni, S.; Cai, C.; Espinosa, R.E.; Osborn, M.; Mulpuru, S.K.; Asirvatham, S.J.; Friedman, P.A.; et al. Efficacy and safety of transvenous lead extraction in the device laboratory and operating room guided by a novel risk stratification scheme. *JACC Clin. Electrophysiol.* **2019**, *5*, 174–182. [CrossRef] [PubMed]
26. Bontempi, L.; Vassanelli, F.; Cerini, M.; D'Aloia, A.; Vizzardi, E.; Gargaro, A.; Chiusso, F.; Mamedouv, R.; Lipari, A.; Curnis, A. Predicting the difficulty of a lead extraction procedure: The LED index. *J. Cardiovasc. Med.* **2014**, *15*, 668–673. [CrossRef]
27. Fu, H.X.; Huang, X.M.; Zhong, L.I.; Osborn, M.J.; Asirvatham, S.J.; Espinosa, R.E.; Brady, P.A.; Lee, H.C.; Greason, K.L.; Baddour, L.M.; et al. Outcomes and complications of lead removal: Can we establish a risk stratification schema for a collaborative and effective approach? *Pacing Clin. Electrophysiol.* **2015**, *38*, 1439–1447. [CrossRef] [PubMed]
28. Nowosielecka, D.; Jacheć, W.; Polewczyk, A.; Tułecki, Ł.; Tomków, K.; Stefańczyk, P.; Tomaszewski, A.; Brzozowski, W.; Szcześniak-Stańczyk, D.; Kleinrok, A.; et al. Transesophageal Echocardiography as a Monitoring Tool During Transvenous Lead Extraction-Does It Improve Procedure Effectiveness? *J. Clin. Med.* **2020**, *9*, 1382. [CrossRef]
29. Nowosielecka, D.; Polewczyk, A.; Jacheć, W.; Tułecki, Ł.; Tomków, K.; Stefańczyk, P.; Kleinrok, A.; Kutarski, A. A new approach to the continuous monitoring of transvenous lead extraction using transesophageal echocardiography—Analysis of 936 procedures. *Echocardiography* **2020**, *37*, 601–611. [CrossRef]
30. Nowosielecka, D.; Polewczyk, A.; Jacheć, W.; Kleinrok, A.; Tułecki, Ł.; Kutarski, A. Transesophageal echocardiography for the monitoring of transvenous lead extraction. *Kardiol. Pol.* **2020**, *78*, 1206–1214. [CrossRef]
31. Nowosielecka, D.; Jacheć, W.; Polewczyk, A.; Kleinrok, A.; Tułecki, Ł.; Kutarski, A. The prognostic value of transesophageal echocardiography after transvenous lead extraction: Landscape after battle. *Cardiovasc. Diagn. Ther.* **2021**, *11*, 394–410. [CrossRef] [PubMed]
32. Morita, J.; Yamaji, K.; Nagashima, M.; Kondo, Y.; Sadohara, Y.; Hirokami, J.; Kuji, R.; Korai, K.; Fukunaga, M.; Hiroshima, K.; et al. Predictors of lead break during transvenous lead extraction. *J. Arrhythmia* **2021**, *37*, 645–652. [CrossRef]
33. Pecha, S.; Ziegelhoeffer, T.; Yildirim, Y.; Choi, Y.H.; Willems, S.; Reichenspurner, H.; Burger, H.; Hakmi, S. Safety and efficacy of transvenous lead extraction of very old leads. *Interact. Cardiovasc. Thorac. Surg.* **2021**, *32*, 402–407. [CrossRef]
34. Mehrotra, D.; Kejriwal, N.K. Tricuspid valve repair for torrential tricuspid regurgitation after permanent pacemaker lead extraction. *Tex. Heart Inst. J.* **2011**, *38*, 305–307. [PubMed]
35. Schaller, R.D.; Sadek, M.M. Intracardiac echocardiography during transvenous lead extraction. *Card. Electrophysiol. Clin.* **2021**, *13*, 409–418. [CrossRef] [PubMed]

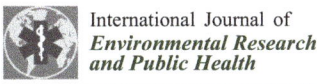
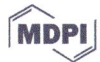

Article

Utilization of Subcutaneous Cardioverter-Defibrillator in Poland and Europe–Comparison of the Results of Multi-Center Registries

Maciej Kempa [1], Andrzej Przybylski [2,3], Szymon Budrejko [1,*], Tomasz Fabiszak [4], Michał Lewandowski [5], Krzysztof Kaczmarek [6], Mateusz Tajstra [7], Marcin Grabowski [8], Przemysław Mitkowski [9], Stanisław Tubek [10], Ewa Jędrzejczyk-Patej [11], Radosław Lenarczyk [11], Dariusz Jagielski [12], Janusz Romanek [2,3], Anna Rydlewska [13,14], Zbigniew Orski [15], Joanna Zakrzewska-Koperska [16], Artur Filipecki [17], Marcin Janowski [18], Tatjana Potpara [19] and Serge Boveda [20]

1. Department of Cardiology and Electrotherapy, Medical University of Gdansk, 80-210 Gdansk, Poland; kempa@gumed.edu.pl
2. Medical College, University of Rzeszow, 35-959 Rzeszow, Poland; a_przybylski-65@wp.pl (A.P.); januszromanek@wp.pl (J.R.)
3. Cardiology Department with the Acute Coronary Syndromes Subdivision, Clinical Provincial Hospital No. 2, 35-301 Rzeszow, Poland
4. Department of Cardiology and Internal Diseases, Collegium Medicum, Nicolaus Copernicus University, 85-094 Bydgoszcz, Poland; tfabiszak@wp.pl
5. 2nd Department of Arrhythmia, National Institute of Cardiology, 04-628 Warsaw, Poland; mlewandowski@ikard.pl
6. Department of Electrocardiology, Medical University of Lodz, 90-647 Lodz, Poland; krzysztof.kaczmarek@umed.lodz.pl
7. 3rd Department of Cardiology, Silesian Centre for Heart Diseases, School of Medicine with the Division of Dentistry in Zabrze, Medical University of Silesia, 40-055 Katowice, Poland; mateusztajstra@wp.pl
8. 1st Chair and Department of Cardiology, Medical University of Warsaw, 02-091 Warsaw, Poland; marcin.grabowski@wum.edu.pl
9. 1st Department of Cardiology, Chair of Cardiology, Karol Marcinkowski University of Medical Sciences, 61-701 Poznan, Poland; przemyslaw.mitkowski@ump.edu.pl
10. Department of Heart Diseases, Wroclaw Medical University, 50-367 Wroclaw, Poland; stanislaw.tubek@gmail.com
11. Department of Cardiology, Congenital Heart Diseases and Electrotherapy, Medical University of Silesia Silesian Centre for Heart Diseases, 41-800 Zabrze, Poland; ewajczyk@op.pl (E.J.-P.); radle@poczta.onet.pl (R.L.)
12. Department of Cardiology, Centre for Heart Diseases, 4th Military Hospital, 50-981 Wroclaw, Poland; dariuszjagielski@gmail.com
13. Institute of Cardiology, Faculty of Medicine, Jagiellonian University Medical College, 31-008 Kraków, Poland; annarydlewska@op.pl
14. Department of Electrocardiology, The John Paul II Hospital, 31-202 Krakow, Poland
15. Department of Cardiology and Internal Diseases, Military Institute of Medicine, 04-141 Warsaw, Poland; zorski@wim.mil.pl
16. 1st Department of Arrhythmia, National Institute of Cardiology, 04-628 Warsaw, Poland; jzakrzewska@ikard.pl
17. 1st Department of Cardiology, School of Medicine in Katowice, Medical University of Silesia, 40-055 Katowice, Poland; arturfilipecki@wp.pl
18. Chair and Department of Cardiology, Medical University of Lublin, 20-059 Lublin, Poland; marcin.janowski@umlub.pl
19. School of Medicine, Belgrade University, 11000 Belgrade, Serbia; tanjapotpara@gmail.com
20. Cardiology, Cardiac Arrhythmias Management Department, Clinique Pasteur, 31076 Toulouse, France; sboveda@clinique-pasteur.com
* Correspondence: budrejko@gumed.edu.pl; Tel.: +48-58-3493910

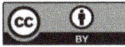

Abstract: The implantation of a subcutaneous cardioverter-defibrillator (S-ICD) may be used instead of a traditional transvenous system to prevent sudden cardiac death. Our aim was to compare the characteristics of S-ICD patients from the multi-center registry of S-ICD implantations in Poland with the published results of the European Snapshot Survey on S-ICD Implantation (ESSS-SICDI). We compared data of 137 Polish S-ICD patients with 68 patients from the ESSS-SICDI registry. The groups did not differ significantly in terms of sex, prevalence of ischemic cardiomyopathy, concomitant diseases, and the rate of primary prevention indication. Polish patients had more advanced heart failure (New York Heart Association (NYHA) class III: 11.7% vs. 2.9%, NYHA II: 48.9% vs. 29.4%, NYHA I: 39.4% vs. 67.7%, $p < 0.05$ each). Young age (75.9% vs. 50%, $p < 0.05$) and no vascular access (7.3% vs. 0%, $p < 0.05$) were more often indications for S-ICD. The percentage of patients after transvenous system removal due to infections was significantly higher in the Polish group (11% vs. 1.5%, $p < 0.05$). In the European population, S-ICD was more frequently chosen because of patients' active lifestyle and patients' preference (both 10.3% vs. 0%, $p < 0.05$). Our analysis shows that in Poland, compared to other European countries, subcutaneous cardioverters-defibrillators are being implanted in patients at a more advanced stage of chronic heart failure. The most frequent reason for choosing a subcutaneous system instead of a transvenous ICD is the young age of a patient.

Keywords: sudden cardiac death; ventricular arrhythmia; implantable cardioverter-defibrillator; subcutaneous implantable cardioverter-defibrillator

1. Introduction

The implantation of a subcutaneous cardioverter-defibrillator (S-ICD) has been increasingly used to treat patients at risk of sudden cardiac death due to ventricular arrhythmias. Such a solution may in many cases replace a traditional cardioverter-defibrillator system with transvenous leads (transvenous cardioverter-defibrillator, TV-ICD) [1,2]. According to the European and American guidelines, S-ICD is contraindicated if a patient requires permanent cardiac pacing, including resynchronization therapy, or has a history of ventricular tachycardia that is possibly eligible for termination with antitachycardia pacing [3,4]. S-ICD systems have been used in Poland since 2014 [5,6]. Due to complex rules of reimbursement, the number of procedures was initially low. Not until the beginning of 2019 has S-ICD implantation been cleared for a full refund by the National Health Fund [7]. To our knowledge, there is no data that compare Poland with other European countries in terms of the population characteristics of S-ICD patients and the indications for the selection of that particular method of treatment.

The aim of our study was to compare patients' populations and indications for S-ICD implantation in Poland with available European data.

2. Materials and Methods

The analysis incorporates data gathered between May 2020 and March 2021 in the multi-center registry of S-ICD implantations in Poland, run by the Heart Rhythm Section of the Polish Cardiac Society without any support from the industry. Participation in the registry did not in any way influence the qualification of patients for the procedure, procedural technique, or follow-up care in any of the centers involved. Data was collected and entered into the registry database when the hospitalization of a patient was finished. Collected information included: age, gender, underlying disease, data regarding indications for S-ICD implantation, basic electrocardiographic measurements, procedural technique, and postoperative course, with any possible complications during hospitalization. Data were compared with the published results of the European Snapshot Survey on S-ICD Implantation (ESSS-SICDI) [8], which collected data from 20 European centers (eight from France, six from Poland, two from Germany and Italy, and one from Austria and Switzerland). Altogether, 429 patients were reported during the period from April to June 2017, and for 383 of them information regarding the type of implanted device was available. In 76, S-ICD was implanted, and in the remaining 307 patients, TV-ICD was implanted. For the purpose of our analysis we only selected data from those 76 European patients with S-ICD but then excluded eight patients reported by Polish centers. Thus, finally, a group of 68 S-ICD patients from the ESSS-SICDI survey was taken for the comparison [9].

Continuous variables were presented as the mean and standard deviation or median and interquartile range, in the case of a non-normal distribution. Categorical parameters were presented as numbers and percentages. The normality of distribution was tested with the Shapiro–Wilk test. The χ^2 test, and the Student t-test or Mann–Whitney U test (depending on the analysis of distribution and variance) were used to compare the groups, as appropriate for a given variable. A p value <0.05 was considered statistically significant. The statistical analysis was performed with the use of Statistica 13.1 software (TIBCO Software Inc., Palo Alto, CA 94304, USA).

3. Results

During the period from May 2020 to March 2021, data from 147 patients have been reported to the registry of S-ICD implantations in Poland, which corresponds to 90% of all S-ICD implantations performed in our country during that time. In that population, 137 patients had undergone primary implantation, and the remaining 10 had undergone a device exchange due to an elective replacement indicator (those 10 patients were excluded from further analysis). Altogether, 15 centers reported on 34 female and 103 male patients (age 15 to 79, mean ± SD 43.4 ± 15.3), the majority remaining in the NYHA II or NYHA I functional class, 67 (48.9%) and 54 patients (39.4%), respectively. The left ventricle ejection fraction (LVEF) in this group ranged between 10 and 80%, (median [IQR] 33 (25–57)). In 91 cases (66.4%), the S-ICD system was implanted for the primary prevention of sudden cardiac death (SCD). Nonischemic cardiomyopathy was the most prevalent underlying disease, with 64 patients (46.7%). The main reason for choosing S-ICD rather than TV-ICD was the young age and long life expectancy of a patient (75.9%). Among patients with an LVEF below 35%, only two patients had a QRS complex width of over 150 ms (nonleft bundle branch block morphology) but were not considered for transvenous cardiac resynchronization therapy because of a high risk of infective complications (one patient had a chronic infection and a history of extraction of a transvenous cardioverter-defibrillator, and the other one had a history of infective endocarditis). Detailed data are shown in Tables 1 and 2.

Table 1. Clinical characteristics of patients in the study group.

Age [Years]; Mean (SD)	43.4 (15.3)
Male; n (%)	103 (75.2)
Sinus rhythm; n (%)	128 (93.4)
Underlying disease	
NICM; n (%)	64 (46.7)
ICM; n (%)	38 (27.7)
HCM; n (%)	6 (4.4)
LQTS; n (%)	5 (3.6)
BrS; n (%)	3 (2.2)
SQTS; n (%)	2 (1.5)
Myocarditis; n (%)	2 (1.5)
LVNC; n (%)	1 (0.7)
CPVT; n (%)	1 (0.7)
ToF; n (%)	1 (0.7)
Primary VF; n (%)	14 (10.2)
LVEF; median % (IQR)	33 (25–57)

NICM—nonischemic cardiomyopathy; ICM—ischemic cardiomyopathy; HCM—hypertrophic cardiomyopathy; LQTS—long QT syndrome; BrS—Brugada syndrome; SQTS—short QT syndrome; LVNC—left ventricular noncompaction; CPVT—catecholaminergic polymorphic ventricular tachycardia; ToF—tetralogy of Fallot; VF—ventricular fibrillation; LVEF—left ventricle ejection fraction, IQR—interquartile range.

Our data were compared with published results from the ESSS-SICDI survey, which after exclusion of Polish S-ICD patients (n = 8), comprised 68 S-ICD patients (22 female), mostly remaining in the I or II functional NYHA class (46 [67.7%] and 20 [29.4%], respectively). In 24 patients (35.5%), coronary artery disease was the underlying disease, while no structural heart disease was reported in another 20 (29.4%). The LVEF interquartile range was between 25% and 60% (median 50%). In most cases (63.2%), S-ICD was implanted for the primary prevention of SCD. S-ICD (and not TV-ICD) was chosen mostly due to the young age of patients—this reason prevailed in 34 cases (50%). The clinical data from the two groups of patients are presented in Table 2.

Table 2. Comparison of clinical characteristics between the study group and the ESSS-SICDI group—Jędrzejczyk–Patej et al. [9].

	Europe	Poland	p
Total number of patients; n (%)	68 (100)	137 (100)	-
Age <18 years; n (%)	2 (2.9)	3 (2.2)	0.7426
Age >75 years; n (%)	0 (0)	0 (0)	-
Women; n (%)	22 (32.4)	34 (24.8)	0.2543
NYHA I; n (%)	46 (67.7)	54 (39.4)	0.0001
NYHA II; n (%)	20 (29.4)	67 (48.9)	0.0078
NYHA III; n (%)	2 (2.9)	16 (11.7)	0.0374
NYHA IV; n (%)	0 (0)	0 (0)	-
Ischemic etiology of HF; n (%)	24 (35.5)	38 (27.7)	0.2674
No structural heart disease; n (%)	20 (29.4)	25 (18.3)	0.0691
Primary prevention of SCD; n (%)	43 (63.2)	91 (66.4)	0.6515
Diabetes mellitus; n (%)	9 (13.2)	18 (13.1)	0.9846
Chronic kidney disease; n (%)	4 (5.9)	16 (11.7)	0.1879
COPD; n (%)	3 (4.4)	0 (0)	0.0133
AF/AFL; n (%)	4 (5.9)	9 (6.6)	0.8493
Sick sinus syndrome at implantation; n (%)	0 (0)	1 (0.7)	0.48
High degree AV block at implantation; n (%)	0 (0)	0 (0)	-
LVEF (%); median (IQR)	50 (25–60)	33 (25–57)	- *
Left bundle branch block; n (%)	3 (4.4)	0 (0)	0.0133
QRS 120–150 ms; n (%)	13 (19.1)	23 (16.8)	0.6798
QRS > 150 ms; n (%)	0 (0)	2 (1.5)	0.3167

HF—heart failure; SCD—sudden cardiac death; COPD—chronic obstructive pulmonary disease; AF—atrial fibrillation; AFL—atrial flutter; AV—atrio-ventricular; LVEF—left ventricle ejection fraction, IQR—interquartile range. Values are reported as numbers, values in brackets are percentages, except for LVEF, where a mean value and interquartile range is given, as marked in the appropriate cells. *—statistical significance could not be determined due to the lack of source data and data distribution from the ESSS-SICDI population.

The comparative analysis showed similar demographic data: the prevalence of ischemic cardiomyopathy and concomitant diseases (except for a higher prevalence of COPD in patients from ESSS-SICDI) in the two analyzed groups. European patients were more often ($p < 0.05$) in NYHA class I (67.7% vs. 39.4%) but less often in NYHA class II and class III (29.4% vs. 48.9% and 2.9% vs. 11.7%, respectively, both $p < 0.05$). The median LVEF in the Polish population was numerically lower (38.3% vs. 50%), but statistical significance could not be determined due to the lack of source data and data distribution from the ESSS-SICDI population. Left bundle branch block was more frequent in the European population (4.4% vs. 0%). Furthermore, in the European group S-ICD was slightly more frequently implanted in patients without structural heart disease, but that comparison did not reach statistical significance (29.4% vs. 18.3%).

Reasons to implant S-ICD and not TV-ICD showed significant differences between the groups. In the Polish group, the young age of patients (75.9% vs. 50%, $p < 0.001$) and no vascular access (7.3% vs. 0%, $p < 0.05$) were significantly more often represented. Additionally, the percentage of patients with a history of transvenous system removal due to infectious complications was significantly ($p < 0.05$) higher in the Polish group (11% vs.

1.5%). On the contrary, in the European population S-ICD was more frequently chosen because of patients' active lifestyle (10.3%) and patients' preference (10.3%), whereas in our group no center declared such reasons (both $p < 0.001$). Anticipated lead-related complications in the case of transvenous implantation were also reported more often in the European group (26.5% vs. 0%). A detailed comparison may be found in Table 3.

Table 3. Comparison of indications for a subcutaneous cardioverter-defibrillator between the study group and the ESSS-SICDI group—Jędrzejczyk–Patej et al. [9].

Indication	Europe	Poland	p
Total number of patients; n (%)	68 (100)	137 (100)	-
Young age; n (%)	34 (50)	104 (75.9)	0.0002
Previous LR complications; n (%)	4 (5.9)	12 (8.8)	0.4697
Previous device infection with removal; n (%)	1 (1.5)	15 (11)	0.0172
Elevated infection risk; n (%)	7 (10.3)	15 (11)	0.8866
Anticipated LR TV-ICD complications; n (%)	18 (26.5)	0 (0)	<0.0001
Preservation of vasc. system for future; n (%)	3 (4.4)	6 (4.4)	0.9915
No adequate venous access; n (%)	0 (0)	10 (7.3)	0.0224
Patient preference; n (%)	7 (10.3)	0 (0)	0.0001
Cosmetic advantage; n (%)	1 (1.5)	0 (0)	0.1548
Active lifestyle; n (%)	7 (10.3)	0 (0)	0.0001
Obesity; n (%)	0 (0)	0 (0)	-

LR—lead-related; TV-ICD—transvenous implantable cardioverter-defibrillator. Values are reported as numbers, values in brackets are percentages.

4. Discussion

S-ICD systems have been implanted in Poland since 2014, yet full reimbursement was introduced five years later. In addition, the sources of further limitations regarding the selection (and reimbursement) of S-ICD and not TV-ICD are still the payer (additional clinical requirements for the reimbursement) and the centers themselves (operators/center experience). At the same time, there are no reports on how such a situation with limited access to technology might influence factors that determine device choice and the clinical characteristics of the population that receives S-ICD. The multi-center registry run by the Heart Rhythm Section of the Polish Cardiac Society established a possibility for comparisons of Polish S-ICD patients with other groups; it also allowed one to compare the indications and reasons behind a choice for a specific device. The results of the 2017 European Snapshot Survey on S-ICD Implantation gave insight into the practices regarding S-ICD implantation in European countries. A comparison of data from both registries reveals some differences between Poland and the rest of Europe in terms of the clinical characteristics of patients undergoing S-ICD implantation and the indications for the procedure. As the source data of the ESSS-SICDI are not publicly open, our comparison is based on the results published by Jędrzejczyk–Patej et al. in 2018, analyzing a subpopulation of the patients from ESSS-SICDI with the exclusion of patients reported to that registry by Polish centers.

The main difference shown by our comparison of the two analyzed groups is the severity of heart failure at the time of S-ICD implantation. In the ESSS-SICDI group, as many as 67.7% of patients were in the NYHA I functional class, whereas in the Polish population it was only 39.4%. Opposite ratios were found for the NYHA III class because only 2.9% of European patients were reported to be in that class, compared to 11.7% in the Polish group. Additionally, the mean left ventricle ejection fraction was numerically lower in the Polish group. The above findings are concordant with those reported by Jędrzejczyk–Patej et al. in 2018; however, their older analysis was based on only eight S-ICD patients from Poland, implanted before the new reimbursement rules were set by the National Health Fund. Nonetheless, the previously observed trends that Polish patients at the time of implantation had more severe heart failure and lower LVEF seem to still be valid. That phenomenon may stem from three reasons. First, as shown by the results of the

European Heart Failure Pilot Survey, Polish patients treated for chronic heart failure on an out-patient basis, as well as those referred to hospitals due to exacerbation of symptoms, had a lower LVEF and higher NYHA class than corresponding patients in other European countries. They less frequently already had an implantable cardioverter-defibrillator in place [10]. Consequently, at the time of implantation, their heart failure was already more advanced. The second reason is that in other European countries the decision to choose S-ICD may be based on such factors as patient's preference, active lifestyle, and even cosmetic aspects (e.g., scar location after implantation) [8]. Due to that fact, S-ICD is being more often implanted in younger, physically active patients, who still remain in good condition and have less advanced heart failure. Reimbursement regulations in Poland do not consider such factors at all when it comes to decision-making on S-ICD implantation. Lastly, S-ICD in other European countries is more frequently implanted in patients without structural heart disease (and, consequently, with a better NYHA class and higher LVEF).

Interesting conclusions may be derived from the analysis of the reasons behind choosing S-ICD instead of TV-ICD. In Polish centers, a younger age was the most frequent reason to select S-ICD, and it was reported in 75.9% of patients. In other European centers, that factor was decisive in half of the patients. There was also a significant difference in the rate of patients with a history of removal of a previous transvenous system due to infections. In Poland, that was the case in over 11% of patients, whereas in the ESSS-SICDI population, it was only the case in one patient (1.5%). Together, active lifestyle and patient's preference were the main reason for S-ICD implantation in over 20% of patients in the European population. In the Polish group such a reason was not reported at all. That discrepancy may be due to the lack of a strict definition of "young age" in both registries, which may bias the rate of that particular indication in either direction. One has to keep in mind, however, that the factor described as "active lifestyle" could have been underreported in the Polish population because cardiologists qualifying for S-ICD implantation who reported "young age" might also have understood other possible meanings under that category that were not specifically suggested, such as "active lifestyle". However, the most important factors possibly influencing the reporting rate of specific indications are the reimbursement regulations in Poland. Current regulations do not list active lifestyle or patient's preference among possible reasons justifying the choice of S-ICD for patients with a general indication for an ICD. That may explain why none of the participating centers in Poland reported such a factor, despite having the possibility to add any additional reasons. We feel obliged to comment also on the high rate of indication described as "anticipated lead-related TV-ICD complications" in the European group. Among Polish patients, no case of such an indication was reported. This may be due to the fact that in our understanding a history of lead-related complications clearly increases the risk of a future repeated occurrence. Therefore, records of patients with the indication "previous LR complications" were not additionally supplemented with another indication of an anticipated risk of repeated lead-related complications.

5. Limitations of the Study

The main limitation of the study is the time difference between data reporting to both registries. The results from the ESSS-SICDI were published in 2018, whereas data from Polish centers were collected until March 2021 and were more up to date. Nonetheless, the introduction of S-ICD in Poland was delayed by several years in relation to other European countries, and therefore the time of experience with the method in a given country from its start to registry data reporting may be similar [11]. The length of follow-up in our registry, as well as the character of data reported so far, did not allow for more extended comparisons of long-term clinical outcomes. Reliability of data in both registries may be another limitation. The registry of the Polish Heart Rhythm Section is being carried on by specific centers, with coordinators prompted to report data, and the appropriate contract is set by the agreement between the specific center and the Heart Rhythm Section. The ESSS-SICDI survey was performed on the basis of a voluntary participation of implanting centers and the use of completely anonymous data reporting. For the purpose of our comparison, relevant data were extracted from the available publication of the results of that registry (a bibliographic cohort).

In most countries, implantation of S-ICD is associated with a significantly higher cost compared to transvenous systems. Therefore, the financial issues and reimbursement regulations might have affected clinical decisions and biased the data.

What is of further note, the Polish registry contains data collected and reported in part during the COVID-19 pandemic. That might have changed and biased decisions in terms of device selection [12].

6. Conclusions

Our analysis shows that in Poland, when compared to other European countries, subcutaneous cardioverters-defibrillators are being implanted in patients at a more advanced stage of chronic heart failure. The most frequent reason for choosing subcutaneous-ICD rather than TV-ICD is the young age of a patient.

Author Contributions: Conceptualization, M.K., A.P., E.J.-P., R.L., T.P. and S.B. (Serge Boveda); methodology, M.K., A.P., E.J.-P., R.L., T.P. and S.B. (Serge Boveda); formal analysis, M.K., A.P. and S.B. (Szymon Budrejko); investigation, M.K., A.P., S.B. (Szymon Budrejko), T.F., M.L., K.K., M.T., M.G., P.M., S.T., E.J.-P., R.L., D.J., J.R., A.R., Z.O., J.Z.-K., A.F., M.J., T.P. and S.B. (Serge Boveda); resources, all the authors; data curation, M.K., A.P., E.J.-P. and R.L.; writing—original draft preparation, M.K. and S.B. (Szymon Budrejko); writing—review and editing, all the authors; visualization, S.B. (Szymon Budrejko); supervision, M.K., A.P., T.P. and S.B. (Serge Boveda); project administration, M.K., A.P., E.J.-P., R.L., T.P. and S.B. (Serge Boveda). All authors have read and agreed to the published version of the manuscript.

Funding: This research received no external funding.

Institutional Review Board Statement: The registry held in Poland has been approved by the Bioethical Committee at the Regional Medical Board in Rzeszow, Poland (decision number 35/B/2020).

Informed Consent Statement: Informed consent was obtained from all patients undergoing S-ICD implantation in Poland. The registry held in Poland only contains anonymized medical and procedural data.

Data Availability Statement: Data are available on request from the corresponding author.

Acknowledgments: In the study, we refer to the published data from the survey on S-ICD designed by the Scientific Initiative Committee of the European Hearth Rhythm Association (EHRA).

Conflicts of Interest: Maciej Kempa—received consultant fees or advisory board membership fees from: Abbott, Biotronik, Boston Scientific, Medtronic; Michal Lewandowski—lecture honoraria, travel expenses coverage from Boston Scientific and lecture honoraria from Abbott; Krzysztof Kaczmarek—proctoring fees from Boston Scientific; Marcin Grabowski—received consultant and lectures fees from Medtronic, Biotronik, Abbott and Boston Scientific; Przemysław Mitkowski—received consultant fees or research grants or advisory board membership fees from: Abbott, Biotronik, Boston Scientific, Medtronic; Stanislaw Tubek—received a consultancy fee from Boston Scientific; Ewa Jędrzejczyk-Patej—received consultant fees from Medtronic, Biotronik, Abbott and Boston Scientific; Radosław Lenarczyk—received funding from the European Union's Horizon 2020 research and innovation programme under grant agreement no 847999; Dariusz Jagielski—received a honorarium from Boston Scientific for a lecture during a webinar; Anna Rydlewska—consultant for Medtronic's Warsaw Education Center; Serge Boveda—consultant for Medtronic, Boston Scietific, Microport and Zoll; Andrzej Przybylski, Szymon Budrejko, Tomasz Fabiszak, Mateusz Tajstra, Janusz Romanek, Zbigniew Orski, Joanna Zakrzewska-Koperska, Artur Filipecki, Marcin Janowski and Tatjana Potpara declared no conflict of interest.

References

1. Rordorf, R.; Casula, M.; Pezza, L.; Fortuni, F.; Sanzo, A.; Savastano, S.; Vicentini, A. Subcutaneous versus transvenous implantable defibrillator: An updated meta-analysis. *Heart Rhythm* **2021**, *18*, 382–391. [CrossRef] [PubMed]
2. Knops, R.E.; Olde Nordkamp, L.R.; Delnoy, P.P.H.; Boersma, L.V.; Kuschyk, J.; El-Chami, M.F.; Bonnemeier, H.; Behr, E.R.; Brouwer, T.F.; Kääb, S.; et al. Subcutaneous or Transvenous Defibrillator Therapy. *N. Engl. J. Med.* **2020**, *383*, 526–536. [CrossRef] [PubMed]
3. Authors/Task Force Members; Priori, S.G.; Blomström-Lundqvist, C.; Mazzanti, A.; Blom, N.; Borggrefe, M.; Camm, J.; Elliott, P.M.; Fitzsimons, D.; Hatala, R.; et al. 2015 ESC Guidelines for the management of patients with ventricular arrhythmias and the prevention of sudden cardiac death: The Task Force for the Management of Patients with Ventricular Arrhythmias and the Prevention of Sudden Cardiac Death of the European Society of Cardiology (ESC). Endorsed by: Association for European Paediatric and Congenital Cardiology (AEPC). *Eur. Heart J.* **2015**, *36*, 2793–2867.
4. Al-Khatib, S.M.; Stevenson, W.G.; Ackerman, M.J.; Bryant, W.J.; Callans, D.J.; Curtis, A.B.; Deal, B.J.; Dickfeld, T.; Field, M.E.; Fonarow, G.C.; et al. 2017 AHA/ACC/HRS guideline for management of patients with ventricular arrhythmias and the prevention of sudden cardiac death: Executive summary: A Report of the American College of Cardiology/American Heart Association Task Force on Clinical Practice Guidelines and the Heart Rhythm Society. *Heart Rhythm* **2018**, *15*, e190–e252. [PubMed]
5. Kaczmarek, K.; Zwoliński, R.; Bartczak, K.; Ptaszyński, P.; Wranicz, J.K. A subcutaneous implantable cardioverter-defibrillator—The first implantation in Poland. *Kardiol. Pol.* **2015**, *73*, 62. [CrossRef] [PubMed]
6. Kempa, M.; Budrejko, S.; Raczak, G. Subcutaneous implantable cardioverter-defibrillator (S-ICD) for secondary prevention of sudden cardiac death. *Arch. Med. Sci.* **2016**, *12*, 1179–1180. [CrossRef] [PubMed]
7. Decree of the Ministry of Health from 9th January 2019, Changing the Decree on the Guaranteed Services of in-Hospital Treatment. Journal of Laws of the Republic of Poland, Issue 77. Available online: http://isap.sejm.gov.pl/isap.nsf/download.xsp/WDU20190000077/O/D20190077.pdf (accessed on 26 March 2021). (In Polish).
8. Boveda, S.; Lenarczyk, R.; Fumagalli, S.; Tilz, R.; Gościńska-Bis, K.; Kempa, M.; Defaye, P.; Marquié, C.; Capucci, A.; Ueberham, L.; et al. Factors influencing the use of subcutaneous or transvenous implantable cardioverter-defibrillators: Results of the European Heart Rhythm Association prospective survey. *Europace* **2018**, *20*, 887–892. [CrossRef] [PubMed]
9. Jędrzejczyk-Patej, E.; Boveda, S.; Kalarus, Z.; Mazurek, M.; Gościńska-Bis, K.; Kiliszek, M.; Przybylski, A.; Potpara, T.S.; Tilz, R.; Fumagalli, S.; et al. Factors determining the choice between subcutaneous or transvenous implantable cardioverter-defibrillators in Poland in comparison with other European countries: A sub-study of the European Heart Rhythm Association prospective survey. *Kardiol. Pol.* **2018**, *76*, 1507–1515. [CrossRef] [PubMed]
10. Sosnowska-Pasiarska, B.; Bartkowiak, R.; Wożakowska-Kapłon, B.; Opolski, G.; Ponikowski, P.; Poloński, L.; Szełemej, R.; Juszczyk, Z.; Mirek-Bryniarska, E.; Drożdż, J. Population of Polish patients participating in the Heart Failure Pilot Survey (ESC-HF Pilot). *Kardiol. Pol.* **2013**, *71*, 234–240. [CrossRef] [PubMed]
11. Lambiase, P.D.; Barr, C.; Theuns, D.A.; Knops, R.; Neuzil, P.; Johansen, J.B.; Hood, M.; Pedersen, S.; Kääb, S.; Murgatroyd, F.; et al. Worldwide experience with a totally subcutaneous implantable defibrillator: Early results from the EFFORTLESS S-ICD Registry. *Eur. Heart J.* **2014**, *35*, 1657–1665. [CrossRef] [PubMed]
12. Kempa, M.; Gułaj, M.; Farkowski, M.M.; Przybylski, A.; Sterliński, M.; Mitkowski, P. Electrotherapy and electrophysiology procedures during the coronavirus disease 2019 pandemic: An opinion of the Heart Rhythm Section of the Polish Cardiac Society (with an update). *Kardiol. Pol.* **2020**, *78*, 488–492. [CrossRef] [PubMed]

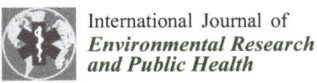

Article

Prognostic Value of Preoperative Echocardiographic Findings in Patients Undergoing Transvenous Lead Extraction

Dorota Nowosielecka [1], Wojciech Jacheć [2], Anna Polewczyk [3,4,*], Łukasz Tułecki [5], Andrzej Kleinrok [1,6] and Andrzej Kutarski [7]

1. Department of Cardiology, The Pope John Paul II Province Hospital, 22-400 Zamość, Poland; dornowos@wp.pl (D.N.); a.kleinrok@wp.pl (A.K.)
2. 2nd Department of Cardiology, Silesian Medical University, 40-055 Zabrze, Poland; wjachec@interia.pl
3. Department of Physiology, Pathophysiology and Clinical Immunology, Collegium Medicum, Jan Kochanowski University, 25-369 Kielce, Poland
4. Department of Cardiac Surgery, Świętokrzyskie Cardiology Center, 25-001 Kielce, Poland
5. Department of Cardiac Surgery, The Pope John Paul II Province Hospital, 22-400 Zamość, Poland; luke27@poczta.onet.pl
6. Department of Physiotherapy, Medical College of University of Technology and Management, 35-225 Rzeszów, Poland
7. Department of Cardiology, Medical University, 20-059 Lublin, Poland; Andrzej.Kutarski@ptkardio.Lublin.pl
* Correspondence: annapolewczyk@wp.pl; Tel.: +48-6000-240-74

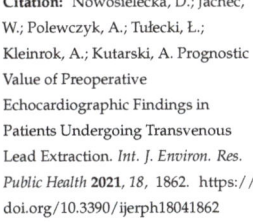

Citation: Nowosielecka, D.; Jacheć, W.; Polewczyk, A.; Tułecki, Ł.; Kleinrok, A.; Kutarski, A. Prognostic Value of Preoperative Echocardiographic Findings in Patients Undergoing Transvenous Lead Extraction. *Int. J. Environ. Res. Public Health* 2021, *18*, 1862. https://doi.org/10.3390/ijerph18041862

Academic Editor: Michael R. Esco

Received: 30 December 2020
Accepted: 11 February 2021
Published: 14 February 2021

Publisher's Note: MDPI stays neutral with regard to jurisdictional claims in published maps and institutional affiliations.

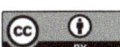

Copyright: © 2021 by the authors. Licensee MDPI, Basel, Switzerland. This article is an open access article distributed under the terms and conditions of the Creative Commons Attribution (CC BY) license (https://creativecommons.org/licenses/by/4.0/).

Abstract: (1) Background: In patients referred for transvenous lead extraction (TLE) transesophageal echocardiography (TEE) often reveals abnormalities related to chronically indwelling endocardial leads. The purpose of this study was to determine whether the results of pre-operative TEE might influence the long-term prognosis. (2) Methods: We analyzed data from 936 TEE examinations performed at a high volume center in patients referred for TLE from 2015 to 2019. The follow-up was 566.2 ± 224.5 days. (3) Results: Multivariate analysis of TEE parameters showed that vegetations (HR = 2.631 [1.738–3.983]; $p < 0.001$) and tricuspid valve (TV) dysfunction unrelated to the endocardial lead (HR = 1.481 [1.261–1.740]; $p < 0.001$) were associated with increased risk for long-term mortality. Presence of fibrous tissue binding sites between the lead and the superior vena cava (SVC) and/or right atrium (RA) wall (HR = 0.285; $p = 0.035$), presence of penetration or perforation of the lead through the cardiac wall up to the epicardium (HR = 0.496; $p = 0.035$) and presence of excessive lead loops (HR = 0.528; $p = 0.026$) showed a better prognosis. After adjustment the statistical model with recognized poor prognosis factors only vegetations were confirmed as a risk factor (HR = 2.613; $p = 0.039$). A better prognosis was observed in patients with fibrous tissue binding sites between the lead and the superior vena cava (SVC) and/or right atrium (RA) wall (HR = 0.270; $p = 0.040$). (4) Conclusions: Non-modifiable factors may have a negative influence on long-term survival after TLE. Various forms of connective tissue overgrowth and abnormal course of the leads modifiable by TLE can be a factor of better prognosis after TLE.

Keywords: transesophageal echocardiography; vegetations; tricuspid valve dysfunction; transvenous lead extraction; long-term survival

1. Introduction

Recently, due to the rising incidence of infectious and non-infectious complications related to cardiac implantable electronic devices (CIED), the number of transvenous lead extraction (TLE) procedures has also been increasing [1]. TLE is considered as a first-line strategy for the management of CIED-associated complications [2,3]. The rate of major complications associated with TLE has been estimated to range from 0.9 to 4.0%, and most often there is damage to the heart or venous vessels; the lead extraction procedure carries a 0 to 0.4% risk of death [2,3]. Due to the continuous improvement in the extraction strategy, most patients with major complications are discharged from hospital in a good general state [4]. Therefore, theoretically the fate of patients after TLE should not differ from those who did not undergo TLE. There is a large volume of published studies describing TLE outcomes, however the results are still unsatisfactory, because mortality is 5–25% at one year, 8–38% at three years, 8–44% at 5 years and 10–60% at 10 years, with the lowest values encountered in patients with non-infectious indications and highest in those with lead-related infective endocarditis (LRIE) [5–23]. Previous studies have not analyzed the effect of echocardiographic phenomena on long-term survival of patients undergoing TLE, and few reports have only assessed their relationship with the risk of procedure. The main echocardiographic parameter considered in order to estimate the risk of surgery was the value of the left ventricular ejection fraction (LVEF) [6,7,12,16] as well as the presence/size of vegetation [7,9–11,13–15,18,19]. Only a few studies based on small sample sizes considered a possible impact of asymptomatic masses on endocardial leads (AMEL) on the length of survival following TLE [24–29]. This paper provides an in-depth analysis of preoperative TEE findings and their usefulness for predicting long-term outcomes of TLE.

2. Methods

2.1. Study Population

A prospective analysis was carried out on data from preoperative TEE performed at a high-volume center during 936 TLE procedures from June, 2015 to October 2019. All patients gave their written informed consent to TLE and analysis of anonymized medical records, approved by the Bioethics Committee of the Regional Chamber of Physicians and Dentists in Lublin no. 288/2018/KB/VII.

2.2. Factors Potentially Affecting Long-Term Survival after TLE

In order to identify the factors that may influence long-term survival the following variables have been analyzed:

Patient-dependent factors: age (during TLE and at first CIED implantation), gender, NYHA class, LVEF, atrial fibrillation, chronic renal failure, diabetes, arterial hypertension, a history of coronary artery bypass graft (CABG), previous sternotomy, CHA2DS2-VAsc score, Charlson comorbidity index, chronic anticoagulation, and antiplatelet therapy.

CIED-related factors: the number of leads in the device before TLE, the number of leads the patient had before TLE, abandoned leads, excessive lead loops before TLE, high voltage (HV) leads, leads in the coronary sinus (CS), dwell time of the oldest lead in the patient, mean implant duration before TLE, cumulative dwell time of the extracted leads, and the number of CIED procedures before TEE.

Indication-related data: diagnosis of LRIE certain or probable with or without pocket infection or only local pocket infection.

TLE efficacy and complications: the rate of complete radiographic success, partial radiographic success, lack of radiographic success, clinical success, complete procedural success and presence of any major complication, hemopericardium, severe tricuspid valve damage during TLE, rescue cardiac surgery.

Most important preoperative TEE findings: tricuspid valve dysfunction, lead-dependent tricuspid valve dysfunction (LDTD), shadowing from the leads before TLE, fibrous tissue binding the lead to the heart structures, AMEL (fibrous tissue encasing the lead, lead thickening, clots and vegetation-like masses), vegetations, excessive lead loops and perforation or penetration of the lead through the cardiac wall up to the epicardium.

2.3. Lead Extraction Procedure

TLE was defined according to EHRA consensus document as intervention with removal of at least one lead that has been implanted for more than one year or a lead regardless of duration of implant requiring the assistance of specialized equipment that is not included as part of the of the typical implant package and/or removal of a lead from a route other than the implant vein [30].

Complete procedural success was defined as removal of all targeted leads and material, with the absence of any permanently disabling complication or procedure-related death. Clinical procedural success was defined as retention of a small portion of a lead (<4 cm) that does not negatively impact the outcome goals of the procedure and with absence of any permanently disabling complication or procedure-related death [30].

Extraction procedures were performed in a hybrid operating room or in an operating room, using mechanical systems such as polypropylene Byrd dilators (Cook® Medical, Leechburg, PA, USA), making use of the oblique cutting edge of the tip to dissect leads from fibrous sheaths that immobilized the lead in the intravascular and/or intracardiac segment [11,28]. Procedures were performed in patients under general anesthesia and after preparation of the surgical field as for subjects coming in for cardiac surgery. Continuous invasive blood pressure monitoring from radial artery was used. The composition of the surgical team and the course of the extraction procedure have been described in detail elsewhere [31–33].

2.4. Preoperative TEE

TEE was performed using the Philips iE33 (Phillips Healthcare, Andover, MA, USA) or the GE Vivid S70 (General Electric Company, Boston, MA, USA) ultrasound machine equipped with X7-2t Live 3D or 6VT-D probes. Images and recordings were obtained before the procedure, after general anesthesia and tracheal intubation, during preparation of the surgical field, and dissection and stabilization of the leads in the region of the device pocket. Leads were evaluated in the mid-esophageal, inferior esophageal and modified transgastric views to visualize the right heart chambers and the tricuspid valve. In order to obtain complete visualization of the structures (and assessment of lead/heart interface) non-standard imaging planes were sometimes required. After the procedure the results were entered into a computer database. The TEE examination was described in detail in previous publications- we followed the methods of Nowosielecka et al. [31–33].

2.5. Echocardiographic Findings Associated with Endocardial Leads: Definition and Classification According to the Anatomy and Characteristic Features

Asymptomatic masses on endocardial leads (AMEL) [31]: Additional masses on the leads classified as clots (varying degrees of organization), components of connective tissue (so-called accretions), masses resembling vegetations (vegetation-like masses), probably the remnants after infections: Old fibrous vegetations or clots (Figure 1).

Bacterial vegetations [31], i.e., multishaped, mobile masses of inhomogeneous echogenicity. Vegetations were diagnosed only if they were accompanied by signs of a general infection (positive inflammatory markers, positive blood cultures) or a regional infection (pocket infection) (Figure 2).

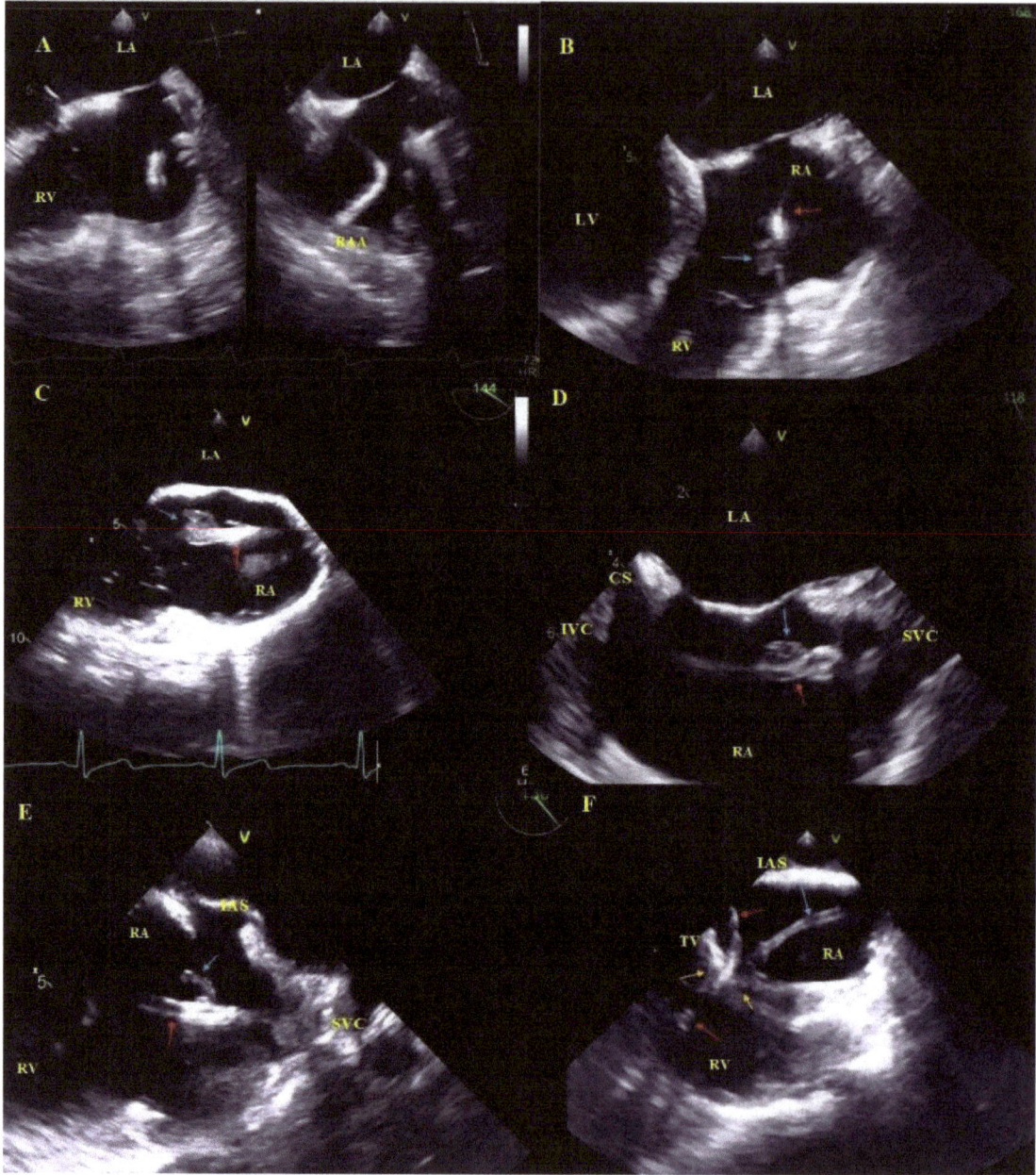

Figure 1. Asymptomatic masses on endocardial leads in 2D TEE. (**A**)—Thickened hyperechoic distal segment of atrial lead surrounded by a connective tissue sheath. (**B**)—Thickened hyperechoic segment of atrial lead (red arrow) with a mobile mass representing a clot (blue arrow). (**C**,**D**)—Ventricular lead (red arrow) in the RA with mobile vegetation-like masses (blue arrow) (2D, ME modified and bicaval). (**E**)—Ventricular lead (red arrow) in the RA with a mobile connective tissue mass (accretion) (blue arrow). (**F**)—The thickened ventricular lead adhered to the TV leaflets, in addition, in RA, the echo associated with the TV (blue arrow) is the sheath of silicone insulation remaining after the first TLE of removing the previous ventricular lead. The place of growth is marked with yellow arrows.

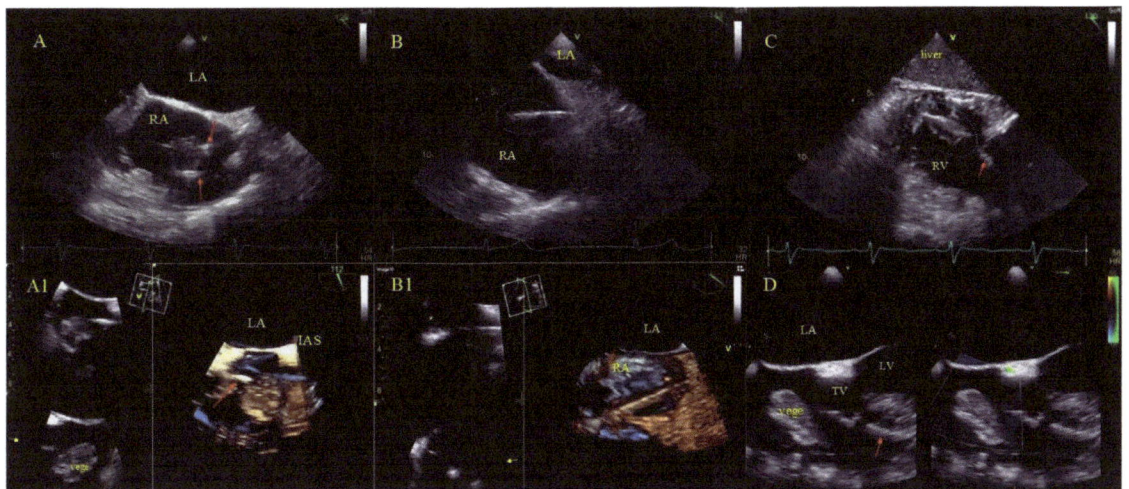

Figure 2. LRIE—TEE images of bacterial vegetations attached to CIED leads. (**A,A1**)—Bacterial vegetation attached to the lead (red arrows) in the RA in 2D and 3D TEE (bicaval). (**B,B1**)—Fine vegetations on the lead causing lead thickening with irregular contour (blue circle) in 2D TEE (**B**)—well visible in 3D TEE (**B1**)—(bicaval). (**C**)—Echoes of the lead (red arrow) with vegetations (blue circle) in the RV (2D, TG, TEE). (**D**)—Large bacterial vegetation attached the ventricular lead (red arrow) dislodging to the TV orifice without significant impact on valve function. The size of the vegetation disqualifies the patient from TLE (2D, 4-CH TEE).

Hyperechoic segmental thickening of the leads defined as connective tissue overgrowth (undergoing fibrosis, mineralization, crystallization and even ossification) [31].

Buildup: Fibrous connective tissue sheath around the lead causing adherence to the endocardium and vessel walls producing images similar to segmental lead thickening but moving along with the cardiac wall. The term encompasses also segmental lead-to-lead adhesion (two or three leads) moving along together with the cardiac walls. Immobile masses binding the lead to the vein or heart wall most frequently represent a sign of pre-existing asymptomatic inflammatory response triggered by the endocardial lead (foreign body reaction). Over time, fibrosis ensues with the presence of calcifications (mineralization, crystallization and ossification). This type of reaction may occur in patients with and without device infections [31] (Figure 3).

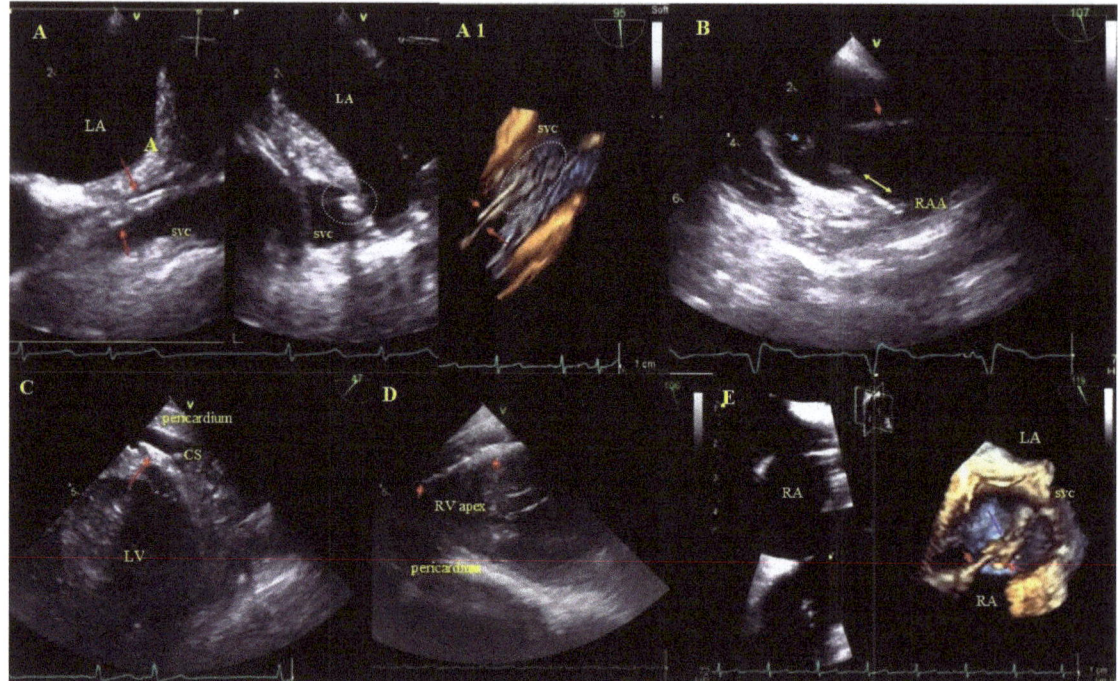

Figure 3. Lead adhesion in various parts of the cardiovascular system. (**A,A1**)—Two leads (red arrows) bound together and adhering to the SVC wall (2D and 3D, bicaval). (**B**)—The end of the atrial lead (red arrow) implanted in the RAA adhering to the RA wall (yellow arrow) and a mass on the lead (accretion) (blue arrow) (2D, bicaval, modified). (**C**)—In the coronary sinus the end of the lead adhering to the vascular wall (red arrow) (2D, TG modified). (**D**)—Long distal end of the ventricular lead (red arrows) adhering to the RV endocardium (2D, TG). (**E**)—In the RA an additional leads (red arrows) fibrous mass (accretion) (blue arrow) at the binding site (3D, bicaval).

Other, separately classified lead-associated phenomena: Lead-dependent tricuspid dysfunction: valve regurgitation (very rarely TV stenosis) unquestionably caused by the lead (lead impingement, lead entanglement with tendinous chords, lead adhesion to the leaflet, leaflet perforation) [31] (Figure 4).

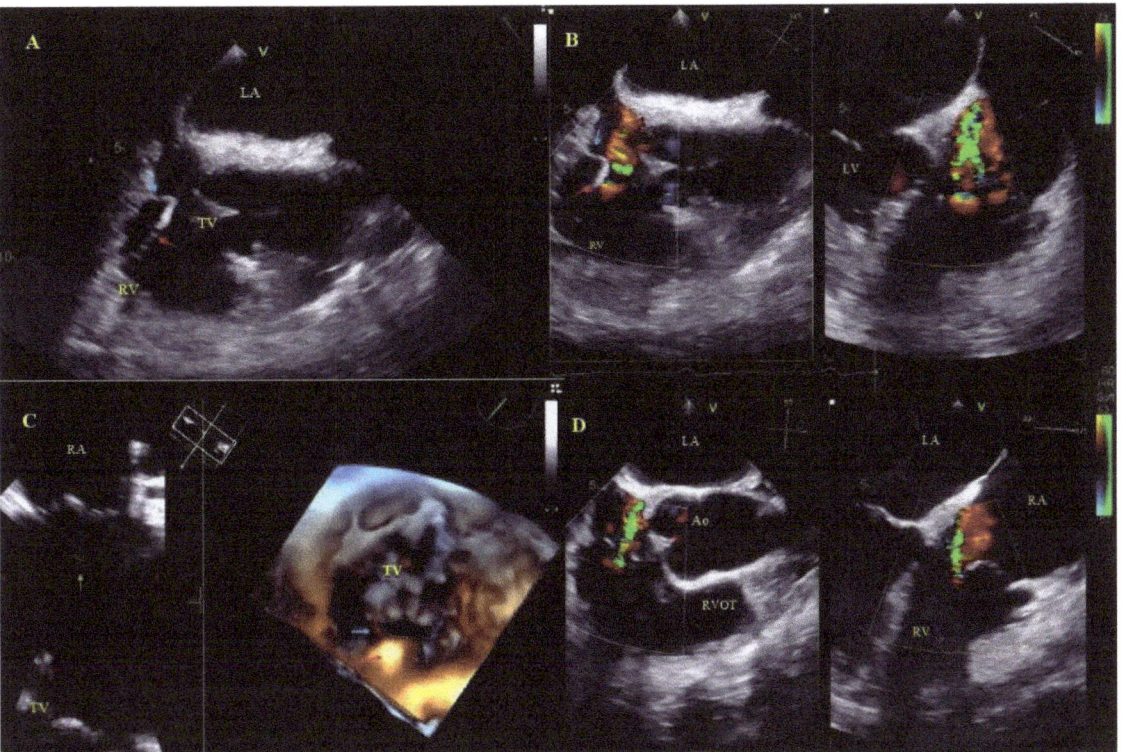

Figure 4. Lead-dependent tricuspid dysfunction (LDTD) due to lead impingement (**A**)—The lead (red arrow) impinging on the posterior TV leaflet (blue arrow) (2D, ME). (**B**)—Color Doppler shows severe tricuspid regurgitation before TLE (red arrow-lead, blue arrow- posterior TV leaflet). (**C**)—3D TEE viewed from the RV- impinging on the posterior TV leaflet (red arrow-lead, blue arrow- posterior TV leaflet). (**D**)—Moderate tricuspid regurgitation after the extraction procedure (2D, color Doppler).

Cardiac wall perforation by the lead: visualization of the lead tip outside the heart contour, frequently with fluid in the pericardial sac; placement of the lead tip close to the border of the pericardium is referred to as penetration (Figure 5).

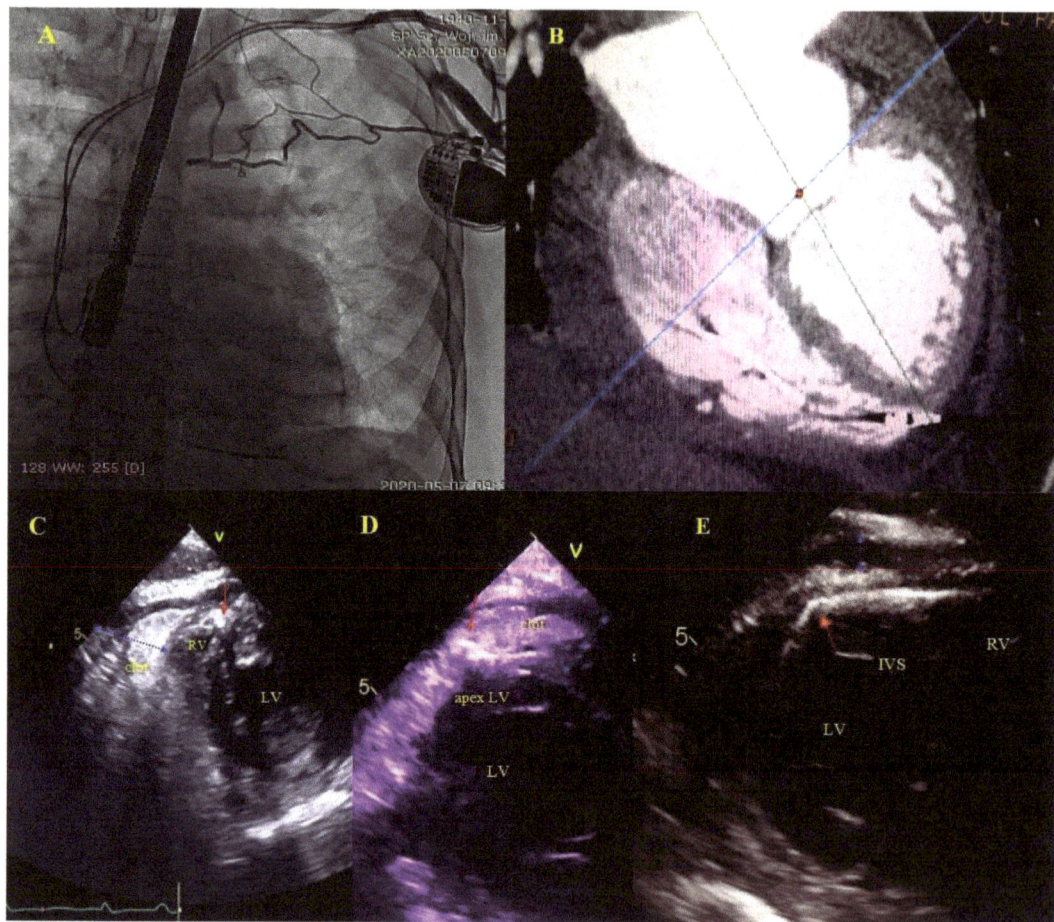

Figure 5. Right ventricular wall perforation by the ventricular lead. An 80-year-old patient with a DDD pacemaker and recurrent pericardial effusion for 3 months. Based on the location of the ventricular lead tip on chest X rays (**A**)—and TEE, perforation of the RV wall was suspected. ECG-gated CT confirmed the diagnosis (**B**)—TEE (2D, TG) during the procedure visualized the end of the perforating lead (red arrows) (**C–E**)—and a clot in the pericardium (blue arrow) (**C,D**).

Excessive lead loops as a result of too weak fixation during implantation or lead fracture with insulation breach in the subclavian region. Excessive lead loops may be encountered in the right atrium or the right ventricle, and in the tricuspid valve orifice (Figure 6).

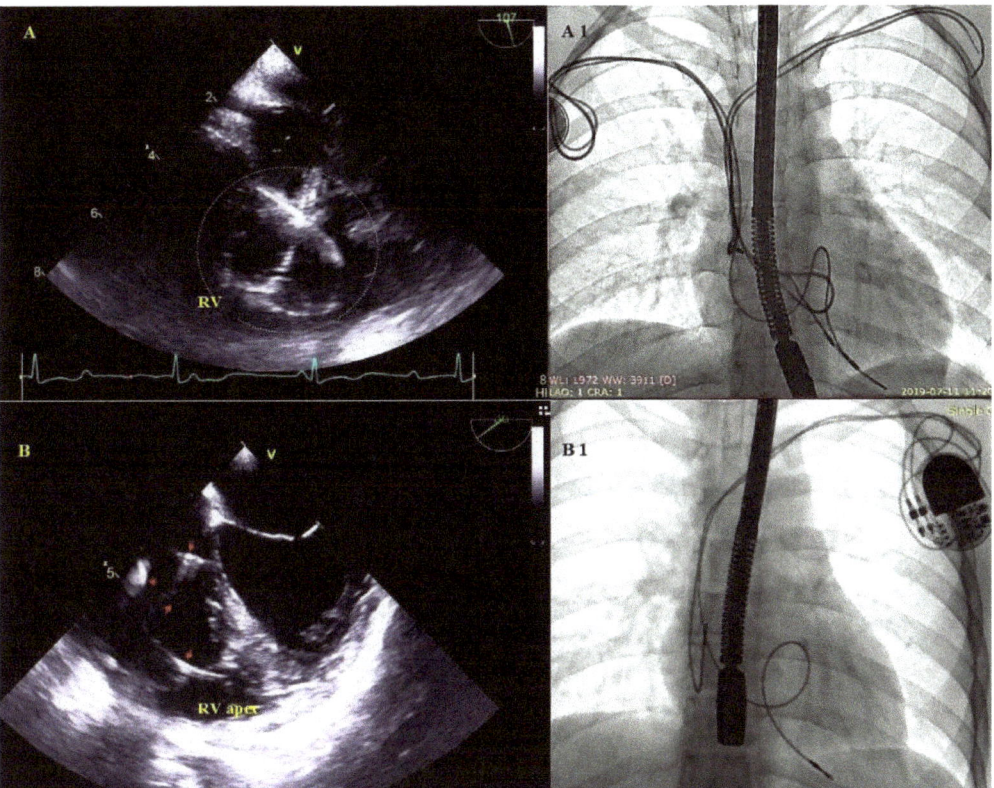

Figure 6. Excessive lead loops in TEE and fluoroscopy during TLE. (**A,A1**)—Excessive loops of ventricular and atrial leads (white circle) visualized in the RV cavity with multifocal lead-to-lead binding. (**B,B1**)—Excessive loop of the ventricular lead (red arrows) in the RV cavity.

3. Statistical Analysis

The Shapiro–Wilk test was used to test the distribution of continuous variables. A non-parametric distribution of all continuous variables was found. For a clearer presentation of the results, all continuous variables are presented as the mean ± standard deviation and some of them (patient age during TLE and during first CIED implantation, left ventricle ejection fraction, dwell time of the oldest lead in the patient) additionally as median with the first and the third quartile. The categorical variables are presented as number and percentage. The study population was divided into two groups depending on TLE outcomes (survival versus death) at two-year follow-up. The significance of differences between the groups was determined using the nonparametric "U" Mann–Whitney test and Chi square tests. The relationship between the echocardiographic parameters and mortality after TLE was analyzed using Cox regression analysis. All variables reached $p < 0.1$ in univariate analysis were included into a multivariate model. Two multivariate regression models were defined. Model 1 was built to assess the prognostic value of the echocardiographic variables only. Model 2 included echocardiographic variables from model 1 and adjusted by clinical parameters of known prognostic values (patient age at first implantation, patient age during TLE, gender, LVEF, NYHA functional class, presence of diabetes mellitus, renal failure, arterial hypertension, infectious indications for TLE, ICD and CRTD prior to TLE). Moreover, the impact of the binding sites between leads and VCS wall and/or right atrial wall and survival after TLE was presented as the Kaplan-Meier survival curves. The log rank test was used to compare the survival distributions of the groups. A two-tailed p value < 0.05 was considered statistically significant.

Statistical analysis was performed with STATISTICA 13.0 (TIBCO Software Inc. Krakow, Poland). All patients gave informed consent for TLE and anonymous analysis of their medical records, approved by the local Bioethics Committee.

4. Results

Transesophageal echocardiography before TLE was performed in 936 patients (355 women; 37.93%), with a mean age of 67.08 ± 14.50 years. The indications for TLE were mainly noninfectious (727 patients; 77.67%). Pocket infection was recognized in 58 (6.20%) patients, whereas lead-related infective endocarditis in 151 (16.13%) individuals. The follow-up after TLE was 566.2 ± 224.5 days (range: 2–730). There were 112 deaths during follow-up. Patients with infectious indications for TLE, especially with LRIE, had a worse survival compared to patients with non-infectious indications: 559.4 ± 266.8 vs. 670.6 ± 167.8 days; $p < 0.001$ (the time of survival during follow-up were calculated for patients with completed two-years follow-up, $n = 612$).

4.1. Prognostic Factors

4.1.1. Prognostic Factors Not Related to TEE Findings and TLE Procedure

Most of these deaths were attributed to patient-dependent risk factors: older age at first CIED implantation ($p < 0.001$), older age during TLE ($p < 0.001$), male gender ($p = 0.003$), higher NYHA class ($p < 0.001$), low LVEF ($p < 0.001$), atrial fibrillation ($p < 0.001$), chronic renal failure (increased, creatinine concentration >1.3 mg/dl) ($p < 0.001$), higher CHA2DS2-VASc score (increased, $p < 0.001$), higher Charlson comorbidity index ($p < 0.001$) and chronic anticoagulation therapy ($p < 0.001$) (Table 1).

4.1.2. Prognostic Factors Related to Implanted Devices

Of CIED-related factors, HV therapy (ICD lead presence) ($p = 0.016$), leads in the CS (LV pacing) ($p < 0.001$) and a higher number of leads the patient had before TLE ($p = 0.029$) were associated with lower survival rates. Similarly, infectious indications for TLE (LRIE) were associated with worse long-term survival ($p < 0.001$) (Table 1).

4.1.3. Prognostic Factors Related to TLE Procedure

The factors related to procedure efficacy and major complications did not affect significantly long-term outcomes after TLE (Table 1).

4.1.4. Prognostic Factors Related to TEE Findings

Of preoperative TEE variables, tricuspid valve dysfunction (degree of regurgitation) ($p < 0.001$) and vegetations ($p < 0.001$) were significantly more common among those who died after TLE. In contrast, the signs of connective tissue overgrowth occurred significantly more often among those who survived: fibrous tissue binding the lead to the superior vena cava and heart structures ($p = 0.024$), fibrous tissue binding the lead to the heart structures (all) ($p = 0.008$), fibrous tissue binding the lead to the RA wall ($p < 0.001$), lead-to-lead adhesion ($p < 0.009$), asymptomatic masses on endocardial leads (all) ($p = 0.022$), and fibrous tissue encasing the lead ($p = 0.021$). Similarly, the presence of (any) lead loops in the heart before TLE ($p = 0.037$) and perforation or penetration of the lead through the cardiac wall up to the epicardium ($p = 0.038$) were associated with better chances of long-term survival (Table 2).

Table 1. Preliminary analysis of all parameters as potential risk factors for early death after TLE.

	All Group n = 936	Alive n = 824	Death n = 112	"U" Mann–Whitney/ X^2 Test
Follow-up (days); mean ± SD; (min.-max.); median, [Q_1; Q_3]	566.2 ± 224.5 (2–730) 730.0 [397.0; 730.0]	604.4 ± 196.0 (64–730) 730.0 [505.0; 730.0]	285.3 ± 221.6 (2–725) 242.0 [75.0; 450.5]	$p < 0.001$
Demographic and clinical data				
Patient age during TLE (years); mean ± SD; median, [Q_1; Q_3]	67.08 ± 14.50 69.20 [61.10; 77.80]	66.07 ± 4.79 69.40 [60.60; 77.40]	73.29 ± 10.54 73.30 [66.70–82.20]	$p < 0.001$
Patient age at first CIED implantation (years); mean ± SD; median, [Q_1; Q_3]	57.28 ± 16.09 60.40 [50.20; 68.10]	56.32 ± 16.45 60.80 [49.90; 68.20]	64.38 ± 10.85 65.30 [59.10; 72.80]	$p < 0.001$
Sex (female); n (%)	355 (37.927)	327 (39.684)	28 (25.000)	$p = 0.004$
NYHA class; (mean ± SD)	2.029 ± 0.574	1.985 ± 0.560	2.348 ± 0.581	$p < 0.001$
LVEF (%); (mean ± SD); median, [Q_1; Q_3]	47.89 ± 15.56 53.00 [34.50; 60.20]	48.97 ± 15.05 55,40 [35.00; 60.10]	39.94 ± 16.96 37.00 [25.70; 55.30]	$p < 0.001$
Atrial Fibrillation; n (%)	219 (23.397)	177 (21.279)	42 (37.500)	$p < 0.001$
Chronic kidney disease (creatinine concentration >1.3 mg/dL); n (%)	230 (24.892)	173 (21.297)	57 (51.351)	$p < 0.001$
Diabetes (any); n (%)	198 (21.154)	167 (20.267)	31 (27.679)	$p = 0.093$
CABG history; n (%)	74 (7.906)	65 (7.888)	9 (8.036)	$p = 0.895$
Previous sternotomy; n (%)	132 (14.103)	116 (14.078)	16 14.286)	$p = 0.932$
Arterial hypertension; n (%)	482 (51.496)	433 (52.549)	49 (43.750)	$p = 0.100$
CHA2DS2-VAsc; mean ± SD	3.005 ± 1.487	2.914 ± 1.763	3.682 ± 1.502	$p < 0.001$
Charlson comorbidity index; mean ± SD	4.886 ± 3.764	4.674 ± 3.751	6.555 ± 3.557	$p < 0.001$
Need for long-term anticoagulation; n (%)	389 (41.560)	323 (39.199)	66 (58.929)	$p < 0.001$
Need for long-term antiplatelet therapy; n (%)	424 (45.299)	365 (44.296)	59 (52.679)	$p = 0.116$
CIED-related data				
Number of leads in the system before TLE; mean ± SD	1.834 ± 0.639	1.817 ± 0.611	1.946 ± 0.745	$p = 0.122$
Presence of abandoned lead before TLE; n (%)	86 (9.188)	74 (8.981)	11 (9.821)	$p = 0.908$
Presence of HV therapy (ICD) lead; n (%)	296 (31.624)	249 (30.218)	47 (41.964)	$p = 0.016$
Presence of CS (LV pacing) lead; n (%)	153 (16.346)	120 (14.563)	33 (29.464)	$p < 0.001$
Number of leads in the patient before TLE; mean ± SD	1.954 ± 0.729	1.934 ± 0.713	2.098 ± 0.718	$p = 0.040$
Dwell time of the oldest lead in the patient (months); mean ± SD; median, [Q_1; Q_3]	115.80 ± 77.6 99.00 [62.00; 156.00]	117.01 ± 77.75 99.00 [64.00; 156.00]	107.24 ± 76.77 84.00 [49.00; 152.00]	$p = 0.066$
Number of procedures before lead extraction; mean ± SD	1.837 ± 0.990	1.840 ± 0.997	1.795 ± 0.922	$p = 0.766$
LRIE certain or probable with or without pocket infection; n (%)	151 (16.132)	108 (13.107)	43 (38.393)	$p < 0.001$
Local (pocket) infection (only); n (%)	58 (6.196)	52 (6.311)	6 (5.357)	$p = 0.854$
TLE efficacy and complications				
Major complications (any); n (%)	18 (1.923)	17 (2.063)	1 (0.893)	$p = 0.632$
Hemopericardium; n (%)	12 (1.282)	11 (1.353)	1 (0.893)	$p = 0.954$
Tricuspid severe valve damage during TLE; n (%)	6 (0.641)	5 (0.607)	1 (0.893)	$p = 0.783$
Rescue cardiac surgery; n (%)	11 (1.175)	10 (1.214)	1 (0.893)	$p = 0.864$
Lack of radiological success; n (%)	6 (0.641)	5 (0.607)	1 (0.893)	$p = 0.783$
Complete clinical success; (%)	916 (97.863)	805 (97.694)	111 (99.107)	$p = 0.534$
Complete procedural success; n (%)	917 (97.761)	808 (98.058)	109 (97.321)	$p = 0.872$

Abbreviations: Q_1—first quartile, Q_3—third quartile, CABG—coronary artery bypass grafting, CHA2DS2-VAsc—Score for Atrial Fibrillation Stroke Risk, CIED—cardiac implantable electronic device, CS—coronary sinus, HV—high voltage, LRIE—lead-related infective endocarditis, LV—left ventricle, TLE—transvenous lead extraction.

Table 2. Preoperative TEE findings and preliminary evaluation of their potential influence on long-term survival.

Echocardiographic Findings before Transvenous Lead Extraction		All Group	Alive	Death	"U" Mann–Whitney/X^2 Test
		936	824	112	
Tricuspid valve dysfunction (degree of regurgitation)—excluding patients with lead-dependent TV dysfunction	Average tricuspid valve regurgitation (0–4 degree) mean ± SD	1.454 ± 0.956	1.413 ± 0.910	1.759 ± 1.210	$p < 0.001$
	Patients with severe tricuspid regurgitation (3–4) n (%)	162 (18.493)	127 (15.423)	35 (31.250)	$p < 0.001$
Lead-dependent tricuspid dysfunction (LDTD)	Average LDTD (0–4) mean ± SD	3.541 ± 0.594	3.500 ± 0.580	3.727 ± 0.647	$p = 0.212$
	Patients with LDTD (any) n (%)	60 (6.410)	49 (5.947)	11 (9.821)	$p = 0.172$
	Patients with severe LDTD (3–4) n (%)	58 (96.667)	48 (5.825)	10 (8.929)	$p = 0.285$
Any shadows on leads	Patients with any shadows on leads before TLE n (%)	607 (64.850)	528 (64.078)	79 (70.536)	$p = 0.216$
Patients with fibrous tissue binding the lead to the SVC and heart structures n (%)		236 (25.214)	218 (26.456)	18 (16.071)	$p = 0.024$
Fibrous tissue binding the lead to the superior vena cava and heart structures	Fibrous tissue binding the lead to the heart structures (all) n (%)	317 (33.868)	292 (35.436)	25 (22.231)	$p = 0.008$
	Fibrous tissue binding the lead to the SVC n (%)	56 (5.983)	53 (6.432)	3 (2.679)	$p = 0.174$
	Fibrous tissue binding the lead to the RA wall n (%)	65 (6.944)	65 (7.888)	0 (0.000)	$p < 0.001$
	Fibrous tissue binding the lead to the tricuspid apparatus n (%)	90 (9.615)	80 (9.709)	10 (8.929)	$p = 0.927$
	Fibrous tissue binding the lead to the RV wall n (%)	106 (11.325)	94 (11.408)	12 (10.714)	$p = 0.953$
Lead-to-lead adhesion n (%)		172 (18.377)	162 (19.660)	10 (8.929)	$p = 0.009$
Patients with asymptomatic masses on endocardial leads (AMEL) (patient analysis) n (%)		437 (46.688)	391 (47.451)	46 (41.071)	$p = 0.243$
Asymptomatic masses on endocardial leads (AMEL) (analysis)	Lead mass (AMEL) (all) n (%)	549 (58.654)	495 (60.007)	54 (48.214)	$p = 0.022$
	Fibrous tissue encasing the lead n (% of all AMEL/% of all pts)	160 (29.144/17.094)	150 (30.303/18.204)	10 (18.519/8.929)	$p = 0.021$
	Lead thickening n (% of all AMEL/% of all pts)	277 (50.455/29.594)	247 (49.899/29.976)	30 (55.556/26.786)	$p = 0.560$
	Clot on the lead n (% of all AMEL/% of all pts)	75 (13.661/8.013)	67 (13.535/8.131)	8 (14.815/7.143)	$p = 0.860$
	Vegetation-like masses n (% of all AMEL/% of all pts)	37 (6.740/3.953)	31 (6.263/3.762)	6 (11.111/5.357)	$p = 0.579$
Presence of vegetations (TTE or and TEE)	Patients with vegetations n (%)	119 (12.727)	86 (10.450)	33 (29.464)	$p < 0.001$
Excessive lead loops	Patients with lead loops in the heart (any) n (%)	181 (19.338)	169 (20.510)	12 (1.7147)	$p = 0.037$
	Lead loops in the RA n (%)	138 (14.744)	128 (25.859)	10 (8.929)	$p = 0.088$
	Lead loops in the TV n (%)	35 (3.793)	34 (4.126)	1 (0.893)	$p = 0.154$
	Lead loops in the RV or PA n (%)	28 (2.991)	27 (3.277)	1 (0.893)	$p = 0.274$
Perforation or penetration of the lead through the cardiac wall up to the epicardium n (%)		151 (16.132)	141 (17.112)	10 (8.929)	$p = 0.038$

Abbreviations: AMEL—asymptomatic masses on endocardial leads, LDTD—lead-dependent tricuspid dysfunction, PA—pulmonary artery, RA—right atrial, RV—right ventricular, SVC—superior vena cava, TEE—transesophageal echocardiography, TTE—transthoracic echocardiography.

4.2. Cox's Regression Analysis Results (Model-1; Echocardiographic Data)

Univariate Cox regression analysis showed a negative relationship between the chances of two-year survival and disease-related parameters only: lead-unrelated TV dysfunction (HR = 1.528; $p < 0.001$) and vegetations (HR = 3.078; $p < 0.001$). However, on the other hand, there was a positive relationship between the chances of two-year survival and the following variables (related to implant duration): fibrous tissue encasing the lead (HR = 0.442; $p = 0.014$), fibrous tissue binding the lead to the SVC and RA wall (HR = 0.208; $p = 0.007$), and lead-to-lead adhesion (HR = 0.484; $p = 0.022$). Additionally, perforation or penetration of the lead through the cardiac wall up to the epicardium (HR = 0.474; $p = 0.024$) and excessive lead loops (HR = 0.543; $p = 0.033$) were suggestive of better prognosis (Table 3).

Table 3. Prognostic value of preoperative TEE findings after a follow-up of two years in TLE patients, results of univariate and multivariate model-1 Cox regression analysis.

	Univariate Cox Regression			Multivariate Cox Regression		
	HR	95% CI	p	HR	95% CI	p
Lead-dependent TV dysfunction (LDTD) (yes/no)	1.630	0.875–3.037	0.124			
TV dysfunction unrelated to lead presence (all) (by one degree)	1.528	1.296–1.801	<0.001	1.481	1.261–1.740	<0.001
Asymptomatic masses on endocardial leads (AMEL) (yes/no)	0.821	0.563–1.196	0.304			
Fibrous tissue encasing the lead (yes/no)	0.442	0.231–0.847	0.014	0.587	0.304–1.132	0.112
Lead thickening (yes/no)	0.911	0.600–1.385	0.664			
Clot on the lead (yes/no)	1.017	0.496–2.089	0.962			
Vegetation-like masses (yes/no)	1.495	0.657–3.404	0.338			
Strong connective tissue scar binding the lead to heart structures (any) (yes/no)	0.624	0.381–1.022	0.061			
Fibrous tissue binding the lead to the SVC (yes/no)	0.414	0.131–1.303	0.132			
Fibrous tissue binding the lead to the SVC or/and RA wall (yes/no)	0.208	0.066–0.655	0.007	0.285	0.088–0.919	0.036
Fibrous tissue binding the lead to the tricuspid apparatus (yes/no)	0.944	0.493–1.807	0.861			
Fibrous tissue binding the lead to the RV wall (yes/no)	0.952	0.523–1.733	0.872			
Fibrous tissue binding the lead to the tricuspid apparatus or/and RV wall (yes/no)	0.886	0.529–1.485	0.646			
Lead-to-lead adhesion (yes/no)	0.484	0.260–0.901	0.022	0.653	0.345–1.235	0.190
Perforation or penetration of the lead through the cardiac wall up to the epicardium (yes/no)	0.474	0.247–0.907	0.024	0.496	0.259–0.953	0.035
Excessive lead loops in the heart (yes/no)	0.543	0.310–0.956	0.033	0.528	0.301–0.928	0.026
Presence of vegetations (yes/no)	3.078	2.042–4.639	<0.001	2.631	1.738–3.983	<0.001

Abbreviations: LDTD—Lead dependent tricuspid valve dysfunction, RV—right ventricle, SVC—superior vena cava, TV—tricuspid valve.

Multivariable Cox regression analysis of TEE variables confirmed the negative relationship between the chances of two-year survival and lead-unrelated TV dysfunction (HR = 1.481; $p < 0.001$) and vegetations (HR = 2.631; $p < 0.001$), and the positive relationship between fibrous tissue binding the lead to the SVC and/or RA wall (HR = 0.285; $p = 0.036$), perforation or penetration of the lead through the cardiac wall up to the epicardium (HR = 0.469; $p = 0.035$) and excessive lead loops (HR = 0.528; $p = 0.026$) (Table 3).

4.3. Cox's Regression Analysis Results (Model-2; Echocardiographic Data Adjusted with Recognized Clinical Risk Factors)

Multivariate Cox regression analysis confirmed the negative relationship between the chances of two-year survival and patient's health status parameters such as patient age during TLE (HR = 1.037, $p = 0.057$), decreased LVEF (per $\downarrow 10\%$p) (HR = 1.168, $p = 0.051$), the presence of chronic renal failure (HR = 1.811; $p = 0.004$), the lead in the CS before TLE (HR = 1.610; $p = 0.031$), long-term anticoagulation (HR = 1.550, $p = 0.032$) and indication-related parameters: vegetations (HR = 2.613; $p < 0.001$) and lead-related infective endocarditis (LRIE) without vegetations (HR = 2.371; $p < 0.017$). But, on the other hand, the analysis showed several variables predicting significantly better TLE outcomes, i.e., presence of fibrous tissue binding the lead to the SVC and/or RA wall (HR = 0.270; $p = 0.040$) and unexpectedly, arterial hypertension (HR = 0.569; $p = 0.006$). (Table 4 and Figure 7).

Table 4. Prognostic value of TEE findings after a follow-up of two years in TLE patients after adjustment of the Cox regression model for common risk factors for poor prognosis, results of univariate and multivariate model-2 Cox regression analysis.

	Univariable Cox Regression			Multivariable Cox Regression		
	HR	95% CI	p	HR	95% CI	p
Lead-dependent TV dysfunction (LDTD) (yes/no)	1.630	0.875–3.037	0.124			
TV dysfunction unrelated to lead presence (all) (by one degree)	1.528	1.296–1.801	<0.001	1.128	0.937–1.357	0.202
Asymptomatic masses on endocardial leads AMEL (yes/no)	0.821	0.563–1.196	0.304			
Fibrous tissue encasing the lead (yes/no)	0.442	0.231–0.847	0.014	0.629	0.323–1.226	0.174
Lead thickening (yes/no)	0.911	0.600–1.385	0.664			
Clot on the lead (yes/no)	1.017	0.496–2.089	0.962			
Vegetation-like masses (yes/no)	1.495	0.657–3.404	0.338			
Strong connective tissue scar binding the lead to heart structures (any) (yes/no)	0.624	0.381–1.022	0.061	1.531	0.841–2.787	0.164
Fibrous tissue binding the lead to the SVC (yes/no)	0.414	0.131–1.303	0.132			
Fibrous tissue binding the lead to the SVC or/and RA wall (yes/no)	0.208	0.066–0.655	0.007	0.270	0.077–0.944	0.040
Fibrous tissue binding the lead to the tricuspid apparatus (yes/no)	0.944	0.493–1.807	0.861			
Fibrous tissue binding the lead to the RV wall (yes/no)	0.952	0.523–1.733	0.872			
Fibrous tissue binding the lead to the tricuspid apparatus or/and RV wall (yes/no)	0.886	0.529–1.485	0.646			
Lead-to-lead adhesion (yes/no)	0.484	0.260–0.901	0.022	0.607	0.313–1.175	0.138
Perforation or penetration of the lead through the cardiac wall up to the epicardium (yes/no)	0.474	0.247–0.907	0.024	0.562	0.289–1.093	0.090
Excessive lead loops in the heart (yes/no)	0.543	0.310–0.956	0.033	0.632	0.350–1.139	0.127
Presence of vegetations (LRIE with vegetations) (yes/no)	3.078	2.042–4.639	<0.001	2.613	1.635–4.176	<0.001
Female gender (yes/no)	0.542	0.355–0.826	0.004	0.812	0.511–1.289	0.376
Patient age at first CIED implantation (↑ by 1 year)	1.040	1.023–1.056	0.000	0.997	0.964–1.031	0.871
Patient age during TLE (↑ by 1 year)	1.044	1.026–1.062	0.000	1.037	0.999–1.076	0.057
Need for long-term anticoagulation (yes/no)	2.172	1.490–3.165	0.000	1.472	0.979–2.214	0.063
LVEF (↓by 10%p)	1.420	1.261–1.597	0.000	1.168	0.999–1.360	0.051
NYHA class (↑by one class)	2.852	2.120–3.838	0.000	1.340	0.909–1.975	0.139
Chronic renal failure (yes/no)	3.528	2.435–5.111	0.000	1.811	1.213–2.704	0.004
Diabetes t. 2 (yes/no)	1.522	1.006–2.303	0.047	1.209	0.780–1.874	0.397
Presence of CS lead before TLE (yes/no)	2.342	1.560–3.516	0.000	1.610	1.045–2.482	0.031
Presence of ICD lead before TLE (yes/no)	1.649	1.133–2.401	0.009	0.930	0.573–1.509	0.768
Arterial hypertension (yes/no)	0.727	0.500–1.056	0.094	0.569	0.381–0.849	0.006
Lead-related infective endocarditis (LRIE) without vegetations (yes/no)	2.289	1.196–4.383	0.012	2.371	1.166–4.821	0.017
Isolated local pocket infection without general infection (yes/no)	0.842	0.370–1.915	0.681			

Abbreviations: RV—right ventricle, SVC—superior vena cava, TV—tricuspid valve CIED—cardiac implantable electronic device, CS—coronary sinus, ICD—implantable cardioverter- defibrillator, LVEF—left ventricular ejection fraction, NYHA class—New York Heart Association class, TLE—transvenous lead extraction.

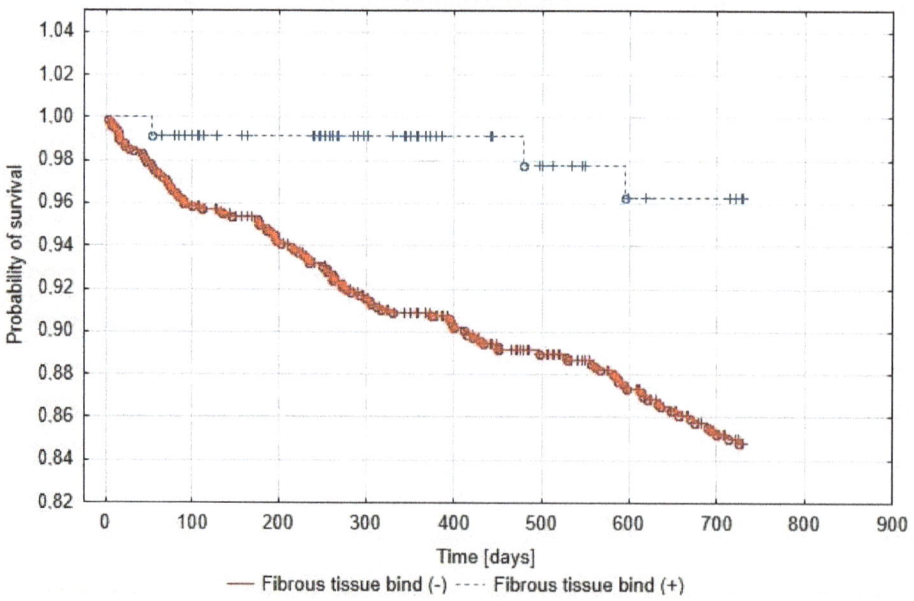

Figure 7. Kaplan–Meier probability of survival after TLE depending on the presence of binding sites between the lead and walls of the superior vena cava or right atrium.

Results of multivariate model-2 Cox regression analysis are also presented in the Figure S1.

5. Discussion

Predicting long-term survival after various procedures, especially those related to the cardiovascular system, is an extremely important element of planning a therapeutic strategy. Transvenous lead extraction has been performed for a relatively short time, and for this reason only few studies have looked at the long-term prognosis of patients after TLE. The available evidence shows that CIED-related infection is the most common prognostic factor for unfavorable outcomes of TLE [5–11,13–15,17–22]. Other factors are mainly those dependent on the patient's general condition i.e., age [6,13,21,22], renal failure [5–8,10,12,13,16,19–22], diabetes [5,16,21], heart failure [7,10,16,22], anemia [8,19], comorbidities [7]. Several studies have demonstrated the significance of procedure-related factors (system upgrade, ICD or CRT device, procedural failure, retained lead fragments, major complications, abandoned leads) [5,6,11–14,16,21] (Table 5).

Echocardiographic phenomena have been very rarely analyzed in terms of their impact on long-term survival after TLE. A couple of papers showed only the role of so-called ghosts, i.e., post-removal, tubular, mobile masses following the lead's intracardiac route in the right-sided heart chambers [15,20]. The present study set out to investigate the usefulness of preoperative transesophageal echocardiography in the assessment of the long-term survival after TLE. The results are consistent with those observed in earlier studies [5–22] which showed that patient-dependent variables (demographic, related to the underlying disease, comorbidities, systemic infection) were the main risk factors for death at long-term follow-up. CIED-related factors, including the number of leads, left ventricular lead and ICD lead play a significant role, but secondary to the underlying condition [5,6,11–15,19,21]. Of the previously identified echocardiographic factors [7,12,16], this study confirms the prognostic value of left ventricular ejection fraction. It should, however be emphasized that the present study was designed to investigate the role of the factors that have not been considered in previous analyses of long-term survival after TLE. Because of the complexity of relationships the preoperative TEE findings and abnormalities were divided into: (1) Non-modifiable factors related to the patient's general condition; (2) non-modifiable factors related to the underlying disease (indication-dependent); (3) factors that have no effect on the procedure course and chances of long-term survival; (4) factors that may increase the complexity of the extraction procedure and the development of complications but which per se do not decrease chances of long-term survival; and (5) abnormalities that can be corrected during the extraction procedure.

Table 5. Potential risk factors for mortality after TLE during long-time follow-up.

Sources			Potential Patient- and Co-Morbidity-Related Risk Factors (Normal Type)			
			Potential Infection-Related Risk Factors (Italics)			
			POTENTIAL CIED-, PREVIOUS PROCEDURE- AND TLE-RELATED RISK FACTORS (Capital Letters)			
Author	Year	Patients	Most Important Factor	Important Factor	New Observation	No. of Refer.
Maytin	2012	985	Elderly pts, *Infections*	Diabetes, renal failure	SYSTEM UPGRADE	[5]
Deharo	2012	197 Inf	*Age, Infection, disease-related factors*	Renal failure	*Thrombocytopenia*, CRT	[6]
Habib	2013	415	*Endocarditis*, heart failure	Renal failure	Co-morbidities	[7]
Deckx	2014	176 Inf	*Systemic infection*, female sex	Renal failure	*Low hemoglobin*	[8]
Kim	2014	80 IE	*Valvular endocarditis & MRSA infection*		*MRSA infection*	[9]
Tarakji	2014	502	*Systemic infection, concurrent infection*	*Renal failure*	NYHA III/IV	[10]
Fu	2015	652	*Endocarditis*	"will be reported"	ABANDONED LEAD(?)	[11]
Merchant	2015	508	LVEF, LEAD NUMBER	Renal failure	PROCEDURAL FAILURE	[12]
Gomes	2016	510	*Systemic infection*, advanced age	Renal failure	RETAINED LEAD FRAGMENT, MC	[13]
Gomes	2016	348	*Endocarditis*		RETAINED LEAD FRAGMENT	[14]
Narducci	2016	217	*Endocarditis, systemic infection*		"Ghost" presence	[15]
Kutarski	2016	2049	EF, NYHA class, AF	Renal failure, diabetes	LACK OF CLINICAL SUCCESS, CRT-P	[16]
Diemberger	2018	169	*Infection*	*Presence of vegetations (TEE!!!)*	Risk factors for development of CIEDI (Shariff score ≥3)	[17]
Diemberger	2019	105 CIEDI	*Endocarditis*	*18F-FDG PET/CT imaging*	*Endocarditis without pocket infection*	[18]
Polewczyk	2016	500 IE	*Vegetation size*, ICD LEAD	*Renal failure*, AF	*Vegetation remnant, hemoglobin*	[19]
Diemberger	2018	121	*CIEDI & pocket infection*	Renal failure	*"Ghost" presence & closed pocket & modified Duke criteria fulfilled*	[20]
Jacheć	2017	1884		Renal failure, age, diabetes, *infection (any)*	ICD LEAD	[21]
Seifert	2018	537	*Staph aureus*	Renal failure, age,	N-terminal pro B-type natriuretic peptide level ≥3000 pg/mL, AF	[22]
Zucchelli	2019	3555	RIATA LEAD OCCLUSION OF SUPERIOR VENOUS ACCESS UTILITY OF POWERED ONES	Notice: only for acute outcome and intrahospital mortality		[34]
Segreti	2019	3555	ABANDONED LEADS	Notice: only for acute outcome		[35]

1. Non-modifiable factors related to the patient's general condition: Tricuspid valve regurgitation (TVR), excluding LDTD, was associated with worse long-term survival in multivariate analysis, but after adjustment for common risk factors for poor prognosis this variable lost its prognostic value. In patients referred for lead extraction TVR is a non-modifiable factor because of right ventricular status.
2. Non-modifiable factors related to the underlying disease (indication-dependent): Vegetations and LRIE have always been (in all previous analyses, including ours) one of the most potent factors decreasing chances of long-term survival [5–22]. Unfortunately, despite the improving standards [2–4] long-term mortality among patients after TLE performed due to LRIE does not improve as desired.
3. Factors that have no effect on the procedure course and chances of long-term survival: AMEL (clots, vegetation-like masses) had no influence on chances of long-term survival in our analysis.
4. Factors that may increase the complexity of the extraction procedure and the development of complications but which, per se, do not decrease chances of long-term survival: fibrous tissue binding the lead to the heart structures, lead-to-lead adhesion. The degree of connective tissue overgrowth in response of the endothelium to long-term irritation by the lead depends on implant duration, stiffness and the number of leads, but first of all on patient age (inverse relationship). This phenomenon has been better documented in papers describing lead removal in children and young patients and in adults with leads implanted in childhood [17]. Surprisingly, the current study found that various forms of connective tissue overgrowth (fibrous tissue binding the lead to the heart structures, lead-to-lead adhesion, lead thickening, scar tissue surrounding the lead) were associated with better long-term survival, although based on previous observations [31,32], connective tissue overgrowth was a predictor of TLE technical difficulty and major complications. This proves that the course of the procedure does not affect prognosis after TLE.
5. Abnormalities that can be corrected during the extraction procedure:
    a. Lead-dependent tricuspid dysfunction was not significantly associated with the length of survival. This can be attributed to the fact that most patients with LDTD were referred for the intervention because of the lead propping one of the leaflets open, which was corrected to varying extent during TLE.
    b. Excessive lead loops (loop in the right atrium, loop crossing the TV, loop in the right ventricle or pulmonary artery) in univariate and multivariate Cox analysis were significantly associated with better survival odds. The reason was that this abnormality was the indication (main or accompanying) for lead replacement and no patient left our facility with abandoned leads.
    c. Perforation, penetration—as was the case of lead loops, perforation/penetration was the main or accompanying indication for lead extraction (most of them were "dry" and caused lead dysfunction or, less frequently, it was an incidental finding or the cause of fluid accumulation in the epicardial space). All perforating/penetrating leads were replaced, thus eliminating their influence on survival and future quality of life. Similar to lead loops, perforations in univariate and multivariate Cox analysis of Model 1 were significantly related to better survival odds.

6. Limitations

The current study is a single center observational prospective study. The lead extraction procedure was performed using mechanical tools and not laser sheaths.

7. Conclusions

The main factors predicting shorter survival among patients undergoing TLE were those related to the patient (patient age during TLE, male gender, higher NYHA class, low LVEF, atrial fibrillation, or chronic renal failure), and those related to the underlying disease, comorbidities and systemic infection.

Non-modifiable factors (patient-dependent and indication/infection-dependent) may have a negative influence on the postoperative course and long-term survival.

The exacerbation of the foreign body reaction resulting in fibrous tissue binding the lead to the vena cava superior or heart structures (especially right atrium wall) seemingly improves chances of longer survival.

Supplementary Materials: The following are available online at https://www.mdpi.com/1660-4601/18/4/1862/s1, Figure S1: Prognostic value of TEE findings in follow-up of 2 years in TLE patients after adjustment of the Cox regression model for common risk factors for poor prognosis, results of multivariable Cox regression analysis.

Author Contributions: D.N.: Writing—original draft preparation; A.P.: Investigation; W.J.: methodology, statistical study; Ł.T.: Data curation; A.K. (Andrzej Kleinrok): Investigation; A.K. (Andrzej Kutarski): Writing—review and editing. All authors have read and agreed to the published version of the manuscript.

Funding: This research received no external funding.

Institutional Review Board Statement: The study was conducted according to the guidelines of the Declaration of Helsinki, and approved by the institutional Bioethics Committee at Regional Physicians Chamber in Lublin no. 288/2018/KB/VII.

Informed Consent Statement: Informed consent was obtained from all subjects involved in the study.

Data Availability Statement: Readers can access the data supporting the conclusions of the study at www.usuwanieelektrod.pl.

Conflicts of Interest: Authors declare no conflict of interest.

References

1. Poole, J.E.; Gleva, M.J.; Mela, T.; Chung, M.K.; Uslan, D.Z.; Borge, R.; Gottipaty, V.; Shinn, T.; Dan, D.; Feldman, L.A.; et al. Complication rates associated with pacemaker or implantable cardioverter-defibrillator generator replacements and upgrade procedures: Results from the RE-PLACE registry. *Circulation* **2010**, *122*, 1553–1561. [CrossRef] [PubMed]
2. Kusumoto, F.M.; Schoenfeld, M.H.; Wilkoff, B.L.; Berul, C.I.; Birgersdotter-Green, U.M.; Carrillo, R.; Cha, Y.-M.; Clancy, J.; Deharo, J.-C.; Ellenbogen, K.A.; et al. 2017 HRS expert consensus statement on cardiovascular implantable electronic device lead management and extraction. *Heart Rhythm.* **2017**, *14*, e503–e551. [CrossRef]
3. Bongiorni, M.G.; Kennergren, C.; Butter, C.; Deharo, J.C.; Kutarski, A.; Rinaldi, C.A.; Romano, S.L.; Maggioni, A.P.; Andarala, M.; Auricchio, A.; et al. The European Lead Extraction ConTRolled (ELECTRa) study: A European Heart Rhythm Association (EHRA) Registry of Transvenous Lead Extraction Outcomes. *Eur. Heart J.* **2017**, *38*, 2995–3005. [CrossRef]
4. Blomström-Lundqvist, C.; Traykov, V.; Erba, P.A.; Burri, H.; Nielsen, J.C.; Bongiorni, M.G.; Poole, J.; Boriani, G.; Costa, R.; Deharo, J.C.; et al. European Heart Rhythm Association (EHRA) in-ternational consensus document on how to prevent, diagnose, and treat cardiac implantable electronic device infec-tions-endorsed by the Heart Rhythm Society (HRS), the Asia Pacific Heart Rhythm Society (APHRS), the Latin American Heart Rhythm Society (LAHRS), International Society for Cardiovascular Infectious Diseases (ISCVID), and the European Society of Clinical Microbiology and Infectious Diseases (ESCMID) in collaboration with the European Association for Car-dio-Thoracic Surgery (EACTS). *Eur. Heart J.* **2020**, *57*, e1–e31.
5. Maytin, M.; Jones, S.O.; Epstein, L.M. Long-Term Mortality after Transvenous Lead Extraction. *Circ. Arrhythmia Electrophysiol.* **2012**, *5*, 252–257. [CrossRef] [PubMed]
6. Deharo, J.-C.; Quatre, A.; Mancini, J.; Khairy, P.; Le Dolley, Y.; Casalta, J.-P.; Peyrouse, E.; Prévôt, S.; Thuny, F.; Collart, F.; et al. Long-term outcomes following infection of cardiac implantable electronic devices: A prospective matched cohort study. *Heart* **2012**, *98*, 724–731. [CrossRef]
7. Habib, A.; Le, K.Y.; Baddour, L.M.; Friedman, P.A.; Hayes, D.L.; Lohse, C.M.; Wilson, W.R.; Steckelberg, J.M.; Sohail, M.R.; Mayo Cardio-vascular Infections Study Group. Predictors of mortality in patients with cardiovascular implantable electronic device infec-tions. *Am. J. Cardiol.* **2013**, *111*, 874–879. [CrossRef] [PubMed]
8. Deckx, S.; Marynissen, T.; Rega, F.; Ector, J.; Nuyens, D.; Heidbuchel, H.; Willems, R. Predictors of 30-day and 1-year mortality after transvenous lead extraction: A single-centre experience. *Europace* **2014**, *16*, 1218–1225. [CrossRef]
9. Kim, D.H.; Tate, J.; Dresen, W.F.; Papa FCJr Bloch, K.C.; Kalams, S.A.; Ellis, C.R.; Baker, M.T.; Lenihan, D.J.; Mendes, L.A. Cardiac im-planted electronic device-related infective endocarditis: Clinical features, management, and outcomes of 80 consecutive pa-tients. *Pacing Clin. Electrophysiol.* **2014**, *37*, 978–985. [CrossRef]

10. Tarakji, K.G.; Wazni, O.M.; Harb, S.; Hsu, A.; Saliba, W.; Wilkoff, B.L. Risk factors for 1-year mortality among patients with cardiac implantable electronic device infection undergoing transvenous lead extraction: The impact of the infection type and the presence of vegetation on survival. *Europace* **2014**, *16*, 1490–1495. [CrossRef]
11. Fu, H.-X.; Huang, X.-M.; Zhong, L.; Osborn, M.J.; Asirvatham, S.J.; Espinosa, R.E.; Brady, P.A.; Lee, H.-C.; Greason, K.L.; Baddour, L.M.; et al. Outcomes and Complications of Lead Removal: Can We Establish a Risk Stratification Schema for a Collaborative and Effective Approach? *Pacing Clin. Electrophysiol.* **2015**, *38*, 1439–1447. [CrossRef] [PubMed]
12. Merchant, F.M.; Levy, M.R.; Kelli, H.M.; Hoskins, M.H.; Lloyd, M.S.; Delurgio, D.B.; Langberg, J.J.; Leon, A.R.; El-Chami, M.F. Predictors of Long-Term Survival Following Transvenous Extraction of Defibrillator Leads. *Pacing Clin. Electrophysiol.* **2015**, *38*, 1297–1303. [CrossRef] [PubMed]
13. Gomes, S.; Cranney, G.; Bennett, M.; Giles, R. Long-Term Outcomes Following Transvenous Lead Extraction. *Pacing Clin. Electrophysiol.* **2016**, *39*, 345–351. [CrossRef] [PubMed]
14. Gomes, S.; Cranney, G.; Bennett, M.; Giles, R. Lead Extraction for Treatment of Cardiac Device Infection: A 20-Year Single Centre Experience. *Heart Lung Circ.* **2017**, *26*, 240–245. [CrossRef]
15. Narducci, M.L.; Di Monaco, A.; Pelargonio, G.; Leoncini, E.; Boccia, S.; Mollo, R.; Perna, F.; Bencardino, G.; Pennestrí, F.; Scoppettuolo, G.; et al. Presence of 'ghosts' and mortality after transvenous lead extraction. *Europace* **2016**, *19*, 432–440. [CrossRef]
16. Kutarski, A.; Czajkowski, M.; Pietura, R.; Obszanski, B.; Polewczyk, A.; Jachec, W.; Polewczyk, M.; Mlynarczyk, K.; Grabowski, M.; Opolski, G. Effectiveness, safety, and long-term outcomes of non-powered mechanical sheaths for transvenous lead extrac-tion. *Europace* **2018**, *20*, 1324–1333. [CrossRef]
17. Diemberger, I.; Migliore, F.; Biffi, M.; Cipriani, A.; Bertaglia, E.; Lorenzetti, S.; Massaro, G.; Tanzarella, G.; Boriani, G. The "Subtle" con-nection between development of cardiac implantable electrical device infection and survival after complete system removal: An observational prospective multicenter study. *Int. J. Cardiol.* **2018**, *250*, 146–149. [CrossRef]
18. Diemberger, I.; Bonfiglioli, R.; Martignani, C.; Graziosi, M.; Biffi, M.; Lorenzetti, S.; Ziacchi, M.; Nanni, C.; Fanti, S.; Boriani, G. Contribu-tion of PET imaging to mortality risk stratification in candidates to lead extraction for pacemaker or defibrillator infection: A prospective single center study. *Eur. J. Nucl. Med. Mol. Imaging* **2019**, *46*, 194–205. [CrossRef] [PubMed]
19. Polewczyk, A.; Jacheć, W.; Tomaszewski, A.; Brzozowski, W.; Czajkowski, M.; Opolski, G.; Grabowski, M.; Janion, M.; Kutarski, A. Lead-related infective endocarditis: Factors influencing early and long-term survival in patients undergoing transvenous lead extraction. *Heart Rhythm.* **2017**, *14*, 43–49. [CrossRef]
20. Diemberger, I.; Biffi, M.; Lorenzetti, S.; Martignani, C.; Raffaelli, E.; Ziacchi, M.; Rapezzi, C.; Pacini, D.; Boriani, G. Predictors of long-term survival free from relapses after extraction of infected CIED. *Europace* **2018**, *20*, 1018–1027. [CrossRef]
21. Jacheć, W.; Tomasik, A.; Polewczyk, A.; Kutarski, A. Impact of ICD lead on the system durability, predictors of long-term surviv-al following ICD system extraction. *Pacing Clin. Electrophysiol.* **2017**, *40*, 1139–1146. [CrossRef]
22. Seifert, M.; Moeller, V.; Arya, A.; Schau, T.; Hoelschermann, F.; Butter, C. Prognosis associated with redo cardiac resynchronization therapy following complete device and lead extraction due to device-related infection. *Europace* **2017**, *20*, 808–815. [CrossRef]
23. Yakish, S.J.; Narula, A.; Foley, R.; Kohut, A.; Kutalek, S.J. Superior Vena Cava Echocardiography as a Screening Tool to Predict Cardiovascular Implantable Electronic Device Lead Fibrosis Cardiovasc. *Ultrasound* **2015**, *23*, 27–31.
24. Lo, R.; D'Anca, M.; Cohen, T.; Kerwin, T. Incidence and prognosis of pacemaker lead-associated masses: A study of 1569 transesophageal echocardiograms. *J. Invasive Cardiol.* **2006**, *18*, 599–601. [PubMed]
25. Downey, B.C.; Juselius, W.E.; Pandian, N.G.; Mark Estes, I.I.I.N.A.; Link, M.S. Incidence and significance of pacemaker and implant-able cardioverter-defibrillator lead masses discovered during transesophageal echocardiography. *Pacing Clin. Electrophysiol.* **2011**, *34*, 679–683. [CrossRef] [PubMed]
26. Strachinaru, M.; Kievit, C.M.; Yap, S.C.; Hirsch, A.; Geleijnse, M.L.; Szili-Torok, T. Multiplane/3D transesophageal echocardiogra-phy monitoring to improve the safety and outcome of complex transvenous lead extractions. *Echocardiography* **2019**, *36*, 980–986. [CrossRef]
27. Golzio, P.G.; Errigo, D.; Peyracchia, M.; Gallo, E.; Frea, S.; Castagno, D.; Budano, C.; Giustetto, C.; Rinaldi, M. Prevalence and progno-sis of lead masses in patients with cardiac implantable electronic devices without infection. *J. Cardiovasc. Med.* **2019**, *20*, 372–378. [CrossRef]
28. Robinson, J.; Wang, W.Y.S.; Kaye, G. Mobile echodensities on intracardiac device leads: Is it always a cause for concern? *Pacing Clin. Electrophysiol.* **2020**, *43*, 388–393. [CrossRef] [PubMed]
29. Dundar, C.; Tigen, K.; Tanalp, C.; Izgi, A.; Karaahmet, T.; Cevik, C.; Erkol, A.; Oduncu, V.; Kirma, C. The prevalence of echocardio-graphic accretions on the leads of patients with permanent pacemakers. *J. Am. Soc. Echocardiogr.* **2011**, *24*, 803–807. [CrossRef]
30. Bongiorni, M.G.; Burri, H.; Deharo, J.C.; Starck, C.; Kennergren, C.; Saghy, L.; Rao, A.; Tascini, C.; Lever, N.; Kutarski, A.; et al. 2018 EHRA expert consensus statement on lead extraction: Recommendations on definitions, endpoints, research trial design, and data collection requirements for clinical scientific studies and registries: Endorsed by APHRS/HRS/LAHRS. *Europace* **2018**, *20*, 1217. [CrossRef]
31. Nowosielecka, D.; Polewczyk, A.; Jacheć, W.; Tułecki, Ł.; Kleinrok, A.; Kutarski, A. Echocardiographic findings in patients with cardiac implantable electronic devices—analysis of factors predisposing to lead-associated changes. *Clin. Physiol. Funct. Imaging* **2021**, *41*, 25–41. [CrossRef] [PubMed]

32. Nowosielecka, D.; Jacheć, W.; Polewczyk, A.; Tułecki, Ł.; Tomków, K.; Stefańczyk, P.; Tomaszewski, A.; Brzozowski, W.; Szcześniak-Stańczyk, D.; Kleinrok, A.; et al. Transesophageal Echocardiography as a Monitoring Tool during Transvenous Lead Extraction—Does It Improve Procedure Effectiveness? *J. Clin. Med.* **2020**, *9*, 1382. [CrossRef] [PubMed]
33. Nowosielecka, D.; Polewczyk, A.; Jacheć, W.; Tułecki, Ł.; Tomków, K.; Stefańczyk, P.; Kleinrok, A.; Kutarski, A. A new approach to the continuous monitoring of transvenous lead extraction using transesophageal echocardiography-Analysis of 936 proce-dures. *Echocardiography* **2020**, *37*, 601–611. [CrossRef] [PubMed]
34. Zucchelli, G.; Di Cori, A.; Segreti, L.; Laroche, C.; Blomstrom-Lundqvist, C.; Kutarski, A.; Regoli, F.; Butter, C.; Defaye, P.; Pasquié, J.L.; et al. Major cardiac and vascular complications after trans-venous lead extraction: Acute outcome and predictive factors from the ESC-EHRA ELECTRa (European Lead Extraction ConTRolled) registry. *Europace* **2019**, *1*, 771–780. [CrossRef] [PubMed]
35. Segreti, L.; Rinaldi, C.A.; Claridge, S.; Svendsen, J.H.; Blomstrom-Lundqvist, C.; Auricchio, A.; Butter, C.; Dagres, N.; Deharo, J.-C.; Maggioni, A.P.; et al. Procedural outcomes associated with transvenous lead extraction in patients with abandoned leads: An ESC-EHRA ELECTRa (European Lead Extraction ConTRolled) Registry Sub-Analysis. *Europace* **2019**, *21*, 645–654. [CrossRef]

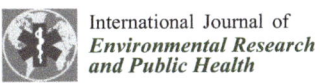

Article

Regional Strain Pattern Index—A Novel Technique to Predict CRT Response

Michał Orszulak [1,*,†], Artur Filipecki [1,†], Wojciech Wróbel [1], Adrianna Berger-Kucza [1], Witold Orszulak [1], Dagmara Urbańczyk-Swić [1], Wojciech Kwaśniewski [1], Edyta Płońska-Gościniak [2] and Katarzyna Mizia-Stec [1]

[1] First Department of Cardiology, School of Medicine in Katowice, Medical University of Silesia, ul. Ziołowa 45/47, 40-635 Katowice, Poland; arturfilipecki@wp.pl (A.F.); wojtekwrobel@poczta.onet.pl (W.W.); adaberger@wp.pl (A.B.-K.); worszulak@poczta.onet.pl (W.O.); dagau@poczta.onet.pl (D.U.-S.); wkwasniewski@op.pl (W.K.); kmiziastec@gmail.com (K.M.-S.)

[2] Department of Cardiology, Pomeranian Medical University, 70-204 Szczecin, Poland; edytaplonska@life.pl

* Correspondence: orszul@vp.pl

† Both authors contributed equally to this manuscript.

Abstract: Background: Cardiac resynchronization therapy (CRT) improves outcome in patients with heart failure (HF) however approximately 30% of patients still remain non-responsive. We propose a novel index—Regional Strain Pattern Index (RSPI)—to prospectively evaluate response to CRT. Methods: Echocardiography was performed in 49 patients with HF (66.5 ± 10 years, LVEF 24.9 ± 6.4%, QRS width 173.1 ± 19.1 ms) two times: before CRT implantation and 15 ± 7 months after. At baseline, dyssynchrony was assessed including RSPI and strain pattern. RSPI was calculated from all three apical views across 12 segments as the sum of dyssynchronous components. From every apical view, presence of four components were assessed: (1) contraction of the early-activated wall; (2) prestretching of the late activated wall; (3) contraction of the early-activated wall in the first 70% of the systolic ejection phase; (4) peak contraction of the late-activated wall after aortic valve closure. Each component scored 1 point, thus the maximum was 12 points. Results: Responders reached higher mean RSPI values than non-responders (5.86 ± 2.9 vs. 4.08 ± 2.4; $p = 0.044$). In logistic regression analysis value of RSPI ≥ 7 points was a predictor of favorable CRT effect (OR: 12; 95% CI = 1.33–108.17; $p = 0.004$). Conclusions: RSPI could be a valuable predictor of positive outcome in HF patients treated with CRT.

Keywords: cardiac resynchronization therapy; dyssynchrony; strain pattern; heart failure; RSPI

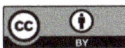

1. Introduction

Cardiac resynchronization therapy (CRT) improves the outcome and reduces symptoms in advanced Heart Failure with a Reduced Ejection Fraction (HFrEF) patients with a prolonged duration of QRS complex, especially with Left Bundle Branch Block (LBBB) [1,2]. Pooled data from six selected studies showed that CRT reduced all-cause mortality by 28% and new hospitalizations for worsening HF by 37% [3]. In the CARE-HF and COMPANION trials, it has been shown that CRT reduces heart failure symptoms by one NYHA class and improves quality of life by 5–6% [1,4]. The main purpose of CRT is to reduce dyssynchrony and to restore physiological activation of the left ventricle (LV) myocardium [5]. A thorough, reliable evaluation of dyssynchrony seems to be crucial in the selection of CRT recipients [6]. The precise measurement of intraventricular dyssynchrony must take into account its two main components—electrical dyssynchrony and mechanical dyssynchrony, which are complementary because the final effect of resynchronization therapy depends on the presence of both [7]. If one of these is missing, CRT is unlikely to benefit the patient. The patterns of the LV deformation strain curves allows a complex assessment of both the timing and contractility [8].

Previous studies have demonstrated that identifying the LBBB-related strain pattern highly predicts the LV reverse remodelling [9]. We believe that a generalized appraisal of dyssynchrony including the analysis of the strain curves from all of the apical views might be a more precise measure to predict the CRT effect. Therefore, we propose a new method, called the Regional Strain Pattern Index (RSPI), which merges information about the dyssynchrony of the strain curves from all three apical views. The objective of this study was to verify RSPI in predicting response to CRT.

2. Materials and Methods

2.1. Population

The prospective study included 49 subjects (84% male, 66.5 ± 10 years, 34.7%/63.3% in New York Heart Association class II/III) with symptomatic heart failure qualified for CRT implantation in class I/IIa according to the 2013 ESC Guidelines [10]. Firstly, 71 consecutive patients were recruited but twenty-two patients were lost during the follow-up (six patients due to poor echocardiographic window, four patients because of suboptimal pace delivery (BiV < 90%), four patients were lost during the follow-up, four patients declined participate in the study, two had dysfunction of CRT (dislocation of LV lead) and two patients died). The remaining 49 patients constituted the study group. Twenty (40.8%) patients had already had a cardiac implantable electronic device (CIED) and were receiving an upgrade to a resynchronization system, while the others (29 patients, 59.2%) received a CRT de novo. All of the patients had received optimal pharmacological therapy before CRT including renin-angiotensin antagonists (42 patients; 85.7%), β-blockers (48 patients; 98%), loop diuretic (46 patients; 93.9 %), mineralocorticoid receptor antagonist (46 patients, 93.9%). The exclusion criteria included acute coronary syndrome for three months, inadequate CRT delivery after the follow-up (BiV pacing rate < 90%) or a poor image quality of the echocardiography. All study patients had transthoracic echocardiography and NYHA functional class assessment before CRT implantation and after 15 ± 7 months follow-up period. All of the patients were informed and signed a written consent. The study protocol was approved by the local bioethical committee.

2.2. Echocardiography—General Data

A full standard echocardiography was performed using a cardiovascular ultrasound system (Vivid 7, GE Medical Systems, Horten, Norway) before and 15 ± 7 months after CRT implantation. LV end-systolic volume (LVESV), end-diastolic volume (LVEDV) and LVEF were measured using the biplane Simpson method. Left Ventricle Global Longitudinal Strain (LVGLS) measurements were performed to assess global left ventricular function. The response to CRT was defined as a ≥15% LVESV reduction after the follow-up period.

The echocardiographic examination included standard gray-scale and color-coded tissue Doppler imaging (TDI) in all of the apical views (4-chamber, 2-chamber and 3-chamber) with six basal and six-midsegmental models of the myocardial velocity curves. Time to peak myocardial velocity during the ejection phase was measured in relation to the beginning of the QRS complex [9].

In addition to the TDI-derived parameters, gray-scale imagining that was optimized for longitudinal strain (with high frame rates; >35 frames/s) and subsequent strain pattern analysis was performed. Two-dimensional longitudinal strain data were processed using a speckle-tracking examination from the apical views and the reference point was the beginning of the QRS complex. The endocardial border was traced in end-systole. Segmentation of the region of interest for a 18-segment model was performed. Segmentation was automatically proposed by the analysis software with visual verification and a manual correction if needed [10].

The ejection phase was defined as the time from the beginning of QRS to aortic valve closure (AVC). AVC was defined using a pulsed-wave Doppler ultrasound in the LV outflow tract from an apical 5-chamber view. The AVC timing was appropriately noted on the tissue velocity and strain waveforms. Three cardiac cycles were taken to average measurements. Echocardiographic images were analyzed offline with a customized software package (EchoPac, General Electric (GE) Healthcare, Boston, MA, USA).

Atrioventricular (defined as the left ventricular diastolic filling time/RR time, LVDFT/RR), interventricular (defined as the difference between the aortic and pulmonary pre-ejection time- interventricular mechanical delay, IVMD) and intraventricular dyssynchrony parameters were evaluated.

The following intraventricular dyssynchrony parameters were calculated:

- Septal flash (0/1)
- SPWMD (Septal to posterior wall motion delay, which was assessed using M-mode echocardiography from the parasternal short-axis view at the papillary muscle level)
- Four-chamber max intraventricular delay—maximal difference in the time-to-peak systolic velocity curves among the four sites (two basal, two midventricular) in the 4-chamber apical view
- Two-chamber max intraventricular delay—maximal difference in the time-to-peak systolic velocity curves among the four sites (two basal, two midventricular) in the 2-chamber apical view
- Three-chamber max intraventricular delay—maximal difference in the time-to-peak systolic velocity curves among the four sites (two basal, two midventricular) in the 3-chamber apical view
- Maximum time delay technique—maximal difference in the time-to-peak systolic velocity curves between any two of the 12 LV segments (six basal, six midventricular)
- Mechanical dyssynchrony index (Yu index)—standard deviation of the time-to-peak systolic velocity in the 12 LV segments (six basal, six midventricular)
- Strain pattern analysis
- Regional strain pattern index—RSPI

2.3. Echocardiography—Strain Pattern Analysis

Strain pattern analysis was performed according to the model proposed by Risum et al. [9]. The pattern of the strain curve in patients with LBBB (so-called "classical pattern") reflects an abnormal, dyssynchronous activation of the LV walls. The classical pattern is characterized by an early peak contraction in the early-activated wall, whereas the opposing late-activated wall is prestretched and shows a late contraction [11].

All three criteria must be fulfilled to identify a strain pattern as "classical" (LBBB-related):

(1) Early contraction of at least one basal or midventricular segment in septal or anteroseptal wall and early stretching in at least one basal or midventricular segment in the opposing wall,
(2) the early peak contraction does not exceed 70% of the ejection phase,
(3) the early stretching wall shows a peak contraction after aortic valve closure.

Strain pattern analysis was performed using all three apical views. If all three criteria were fulfilled in at least one view, then the strain pattern was recognized as being "classical". A pattern that did not fulfill the criteria of a classical pattern was considered to be a "heterogeneous pattern".

2.4. Echocardiography—Regional Strain Pattern Index

Our innovative scoring system is based on the methodology of strain pattern analysis that was proposed by Risum et al. [9]. By definition, the classical pattern includes three criteria, but it comprises four components, actually: (1) the early contraction of the early-activated wall, (2) the prestretching of the opposing, late-activated wall, (3) the contraction of the early-activated wall occurs in the first 70% of the systolic ejection phase and (4) the peak contraction of the late-activated wall occurs after aortic valve closure. Illustration of the four components of RSPI is shown on Figure 1.

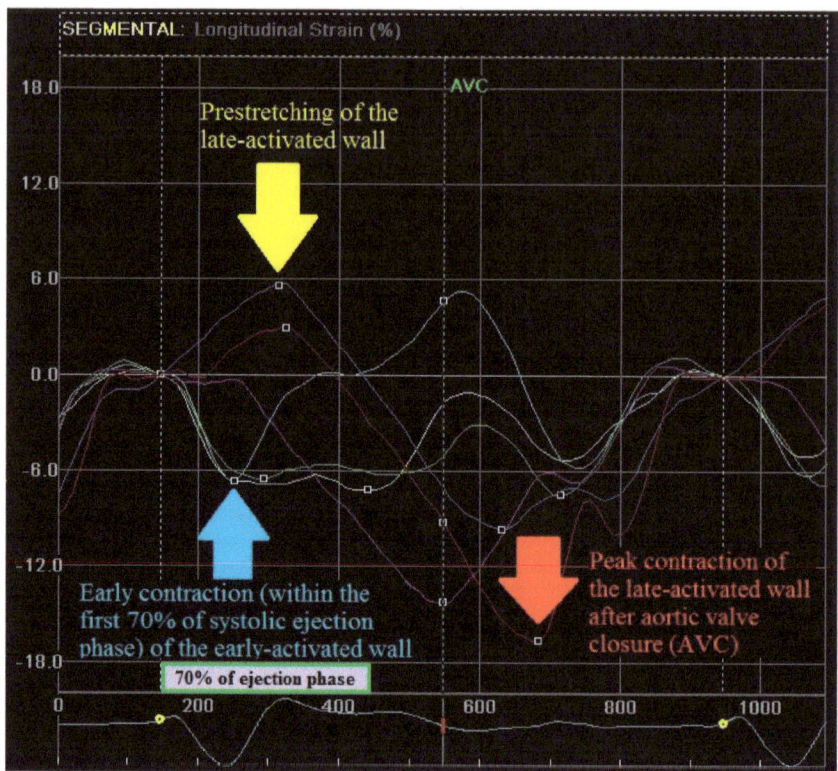

Figure 1. Components of Regional Strain Pattern Index (RSPI). Illustration of the four components of RSPI based on an analysis of the 4-chamber apical view strain curves: (1) the early contraction of the early-activated wall (light blue line; light blue arrow); (2) the prestretching of the opposing, late-activated wall (blue line, yellow arrow); (3) the contraction of the early-activated wall occurs in the first 70% of the systolic ejection phase and (4) the peak contraction of the late-activated wall occurs after aortic valve closure (red line, red arrow). AVC indicates aortic valve closure.

The component "contraction of the early-activated wall within the first 70% of the systolic ejection phase" was verified based on the timing measurements (time to peak systolic strain of the early activated wall with regard to the ejection phase time). The remaining three components were based on a visual assessment and were referred to as peak strain curve. The presence of RSPI component was recognized if there was an evident positive/negative peak strain curve. Evaluation of echo strain measurements was performed by one observer. In 20 randomly selected strain studies the inter- and intra-observer variabilities for the longitudinal strain were 7 and 5%, respectively.

RSPI calculation is based on strain curves analysis from apical 4-, 2-, and 3-chamber views. RSPI was calculated as the sum of dyssynchronous components from all three apical views. One point was attributed to the presence of each component, thus a maximum of 12 points could be achieved (four points in each view). Presence of dyssynchronous components was analyzed among basal or midventricular segments. RSPI has no relation to the type of strain pattern (classical or heterogeneous). An example how to calculate RSPI is shown in Figures 2–4.

The study population was divided into two groups according to the RSPI score: ≥7 points (19 patients, 38.8% of the population) and <7 points (30 patients, 61.2% of the population).

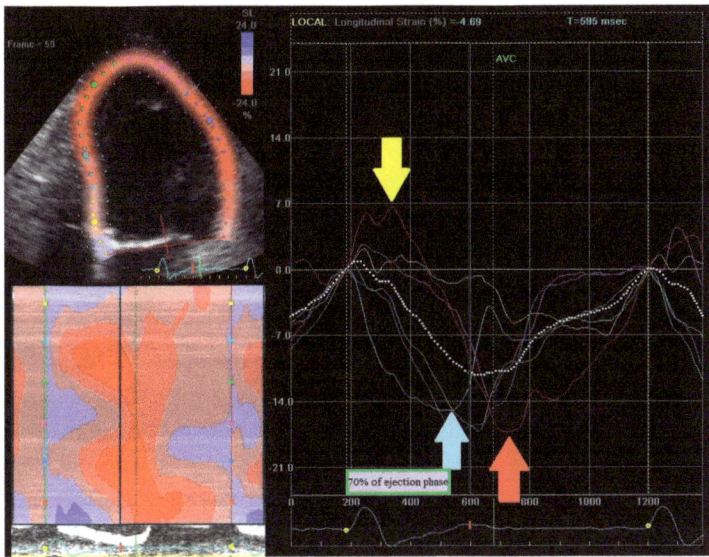

Figure 2. RSPI calculation: 4-chamber view. In 4-chamber view patient reached 3 points: early contraction of the midventricular segment (light blue line; light blue arrow) in the interventricular septum [1 point] but peak contraction slightly exceeds 70% of the systolic ejection phase [0 point]; early prestretching of the basal segment (red line; yellow arrow) in the lateral wall [1 point] with the peak contraction (red arrow) after aortic valve closure [1 point].

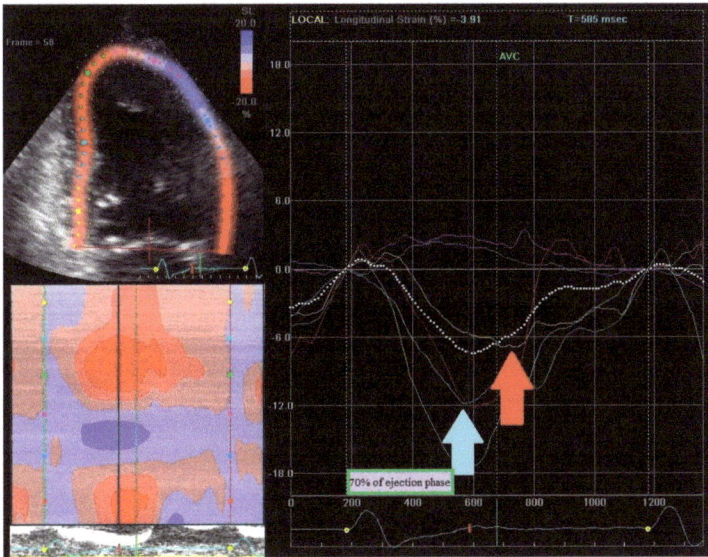

Figure 3. RSPI calculation: 2-chamber view. In 2-chamber view patient reached 2 point: the basal segment in the anterior wall exhibits contraction movement (red line; light blue arrow) [1 point], but it does not fulfill criterion of early 70% of the ejection phase [0 point]. The basal segment in the inferior wall (yellow line) does not show early stretching [0 point] but peak contraction occurs after aortic valve closure (red arrow) [1 point].

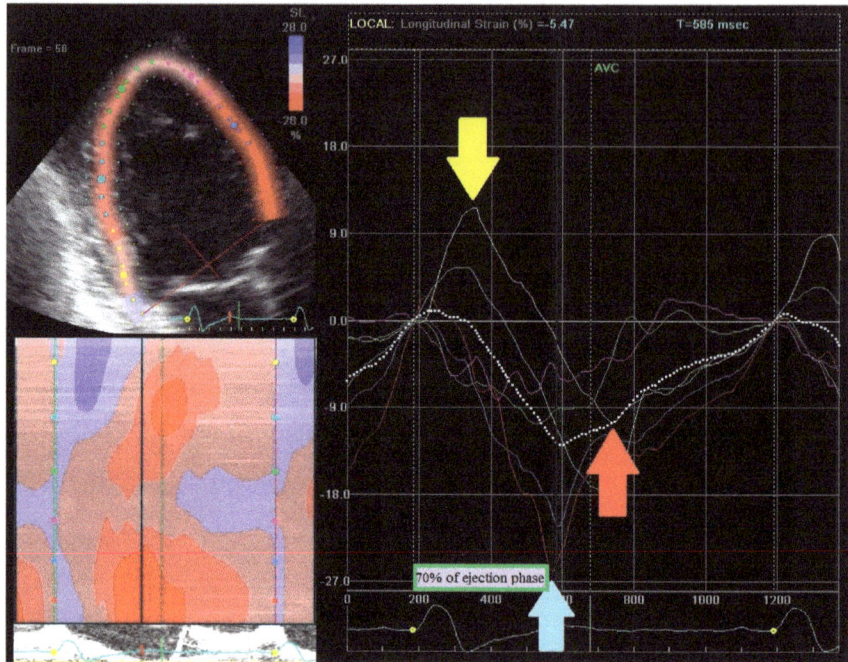

Figure 4. RSPI calculation: 3-chamber view. In 3-chamber view patient reached 3 points: early contraction of the basal segment (red line; light blue arrow) in the anteroseptal wall [1 point] but peak contraction exceeds 70% of the systolic ejection phase [0 point]; early prestretching of the basal segment (yellow line; yellow arrow) in the posterior wall [1 point] with the peak contraction (red arrow) after aortic valve closure [1 point].

2.5. Statistical Analysis

The statistical analysis was performed using Statistica 10 Software. The distribution was verified using a Shapiro-Wilk test. Continuous variables were compared using Kolmogorov-Smirnov test or Wilcoxon test when appropriate. The comparison of RSPI score between groups was performed by Mann-Whitney U test. Categorical variables (reported as numbers with percentages) were tested using χ^2 statistics and the McNemar test when appropriate. Spearman rank coefficients tests were used to determine the relationships between the variables. Univariate regression analysis with dyssynchrony indexes as the independent variables was also performed. The receiver operating characteristics (ROC) was analyzed for RSPI. Reproducibility was assessed for the strain measurements. p value < 0.05 was considered to be statistically significant.

3. Results

3.1. Baseline Characteristics

The study included 49 patients (84% male, 66.5 ± 10 years, NYHA II/III/IV: 34.7%/63.3%/2%; 57.1% ischemic etiology of HF), who underwent CRT implantation. The mean QRS duration was 173.1 ± 19.1 ms. Thirty-five (71.4%) patients had a native LBBB according to the ESC 2013 criteria. Seven (14.3%) patients had a dominant right ventricular pacing rhythm (pacemaker-dependent patients, and therefore native rhythm could not be defined) and seven patients had a non-LBBB morphology. Twenty (40.8%) patients had CIED (three pacemakers (PM) and 17 ICD) and underwent an upgrade to a resynchronization system. Among the three patients with a previously implanted PM, two had a dominant right ventricular pacing rhythm and one had LBBB. Among the 17 patients with ICD, five of them had a dominant right ventricular pacing rhythm, 10 had LBBB and two had non-LBBB. Thirty-two (65.3%) patients had a contraction pattern (classical pattern) that was typical for LBBB and 17 (34.7%) patients had a heterogeneous pattern according to Risum's method. The baseline characteristics are presented in Table 1. Thirty-six (73.5%) patients responded positively to CRT. No significant differences between responders and non-responders were observed regarding baseline demographics, clinical or echocardiographic parameters. However, non-responders compared with responders were more likely to have CIED before CRT implantation and they underwent "up-grade to CRT" (not de novo implantation).

Table 1. Baseline characteristics of general population, responders and non-responders.

	Study Population ($n = 49$)	Responders ($n = 36$)	Non-Responders ($n = 13$)
Age (years)	67 ± 10	68 ± 10	63 ± 10
Male Sex, n (%)	41 (84)	30 (83.3)	11 (84.6)
NYHA Functional Class	2.8 ± 0.5	2.8 ± 0.6	2.7 ± 0.4
Baseline NYHA Class III, n (%)	31 (63.3)	21 (58.3)	10 (76.9)
Ischemic Etiology of HF, n (%)	28 (57.1)	20 (55.6)	8 (61.5)
QRS (ms)	173 ± 19	173 ± 21	174 ± 16
LBBB, n (%)	35 (71.4)	27 (75)	8 (61.5)
AF at Implantation, n (%)	7 (14.3)	6 (16.7)	1 (7.7)
CIED Before CRT (= up-grade to CRT), n (%) *	20 (40.8)	11 (30.6)	9 (69.2)
LVESV (mL)	218 ± 109	217 ± 107	223 ± 119
LVEF (%)	25 ± 6	24 ± 6	27 ± 7

Note: NYHA: New York Heart Association; HF: Heart Failure; QRS = QRS width; LBBB—Left Bundle Branch Block; AF: Atrial Fibrillation; CIED: Cardiac Implantable Electronic Device; CRT: Cardiac Resynchronization Therapy; LVESV: Left Ventricular Ventricular End Systolic Volume; LVEF: Left Ventricular Ejection Fraction; * $p < 0.05$ responders vs non-responders.

3.2. Follow-Up

The mean follow-up was 14.9 ± 7 months. For the entire study group, a significant decrease in NYHA class was observed (from 2.75 ± 0.52 to 1.9 ± 0.7; $p < 0.001$). There were no important differences in the clinical response between the responders and non-responders (Table 2). During the follow-up, almost all of the echocardiographic parameters improved. The LVEDV and LVESV volumes were reduced. The LVEF increased from 24.9 ± 6.4% to 31.9 ± 6.9%; $p < 0.001$. LVGLS) for the entire population increased from −6.94 ± 2.16 to −7.95 ± 2.68%; $p = 0.039$.

3.3. Effect of CRT on the Dyssynchrony Parameters

Table 2 shows the changes in dyssynchrony indexes after CRT. All of the fields of dyssynchrony improved after CRT implantation. The incidence of the septal flash and the typical LBBB contraction pattern decreased (from 31.1% to 11.1%, $p = 0.039$ and from 65.3% to 12.2%, $p < 0.001$, respectively). Similarly, tissue velocity—derived dyssynchrony indexes changed significantly after CRT. A significant reduction of dyssynchrony was observed in the responders but not in the non-responder group.

3.4. Regional Strain Pattern Index

The RSPI was higher in the responders than in the non-responders (5.86 ± 2.92 vs. 4.08 ± 2.4; $p = 0.044$). The RSPI was independent of gender (male: 5.15 ± 2.93; female: 6.63 ± 2.34; $p = 0.21$), HF etiology (ischemic vs. non-ischemic: 5.18 ± 2.83 vs. 5.67 ± 2.99, respectively; $p = 0.72$) or the presence of LBBB (LBBB: 5.83 ± 2.68; non-LBBB 4.29 ± 3.15; $p = 0.15$). No correlation was found between the RSPI and the echocardiography parameters, dyssynchrony indexes, QRS duration or NYHA class.

Table 2. Dyssynchrony indexes and NYHA class before and after CRT in responders and non-responders.

	Responders			Non-Responders		
	Baseline	After CRT	p Value	Baseline	After CRT	p Value
Echocardiographic Parameters						
LVEF (%)	24 ± 6	34 ± 7	<0.001	27 ± 7	27 ± 5	0.433
LVESV (mL)	217 ± 107	147 ± 87	<0.001	223 ± 119	218 ± 110	0.6
LVEDV (mL)	277 ± 127	218 ± 107	<0.001	298 ± 139	294 ± 142	0.35
Dyssynchrony Indexes						
LVDFT/RR (%)	40.5 ± 9	49.3 ± 6.6	<0.001	43.5 ± 9.5	43.8 ± 8.2	0.753
Interventricular Mechanical Delay (IVMD) (ms)	36.7 ± 36	13.2 ± 19.5	<0.001	36.9 ± 31.7	14.6 ± 22	0.025
Septal Flash, n (%)	11 (32.4)	2 (5.9)	0.016	3 (27.3)	3 (27.3)	0.617
SPWMD (ms)	82.3 ± 176.5	−44.3 ± 101.2	0.002	85.4 ± 116	20 ± 194.4	0.424
4-chamber Max Intraventricular Delay (ms)	99.2 ± 80.5	100.6 ± 84.8	0.812	123.8 ± 101.5	108.3 ± 137.4	0.456
Maximum Time Delay Technique (ms)	168.3 ± 107.7	137.8 ± 74.8	0.164	204.6 ± 93	162.5 ± 113.7	0.196
Maximal Opposing Wall Delay (ms)	144.7 ± 94.3	123.3 ± 76.5	0.21	177.7 ± 92	139.2 ± 117.2	0.21
Yu Index (ms)	60.1 ± 40.6	46.9 ± 24.3	0.109	71.6 ± 34.4	53.8 ± 31.2	0.158
Classical Pattern (0/1), n (%)	11/25 (30.6/69.4)	32/4 (88.9/11.1)	<0.001 (McNemar's test)	6/7 (46.2/53.8)	11/2 (84.6/15.4)	0.13 (McNemar's test)
RSPI	5.86 ± 2.9	2.69 ± 2.3	<0.001	4.08 ± 2.4	2.31 ± 2.2	0.083
Clinical Response						
NYHA Class	2.8 ± 0.6	1.9 ± 0.7	<0.0001	2.7 ± 0.4	2 ± 0.7	0.005

Note: LVEF: Left Ventricular Ejection Fraction; LVESV: Left Ventricular Ventricular End Systolic Volume; LVEDV: Left Ventricular Ventricular End Diastolic Volume; LVDFT/RR: Left Ventricular Diastolic Filling Time/RR ratio: SPWMD Septal-To-Posterior Wall Motion Delay; RSPI: Regional Strain Pattern Index; NYHA: New York Heart Association; CRT: Cardiac Resynchronization Therapy.

ROC curve analysis was performed for the RSPI (Figure 5). The optimal cut-off value to predict CRT response was at 7 points. RSPI ≥ 7 had a 50% sensitivity, a 92% specificity and a 64.7% positive and 40% negative predictive value in predicting the CRT response (area under curve, AUC = 0.691, p = 0.014).

In the RSPI ≥ 7 points group, reverse remodelling (defined as a reduction of LVESV ≥ 15%) was observed in 18/19 patients (94.7%). Among the non-responders, only one patient (1/13; 7.7%) had RSPI of more than seven points and the other 12 patients (92.3%) were in the RSPI < 7 points group (p < 0.01).

3.5. Prediction of the Response to CRT

At the 15-month follow-up, the mean LVESV reduction was 23.2 ± 19.8 % (range −22% to 72.3%). None of the baseline dyssynchrony indices correlated with the LVESV reduction. For the entire population, the RSPI did not show a relationship with the reverse remodelling (rho = 0.079; p = 0.59). In the univariate logistic regression analysis (Table 3) among all of the dyssynchrony indexes, only the RSPI ≥ 7 points predicted a positive response to CRT (OR: 12; 95% CI = 1.33–108.17; p = 0.027).

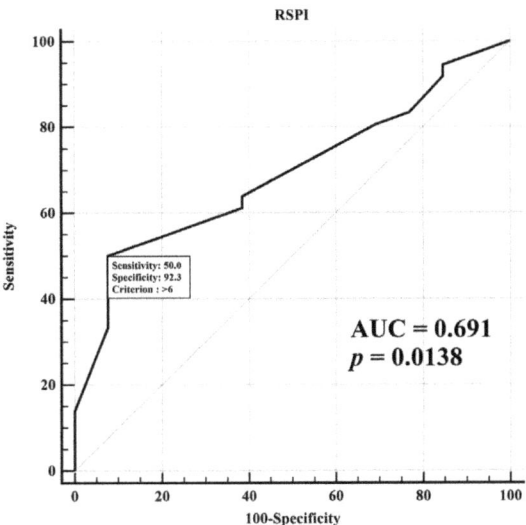

Figure 5. Receiver operating characteristic curves for Regional Strain Pattern Index (RSPI) in prediction of Cardiac Resynchronization Therapy (CRT) response (AUC = area under the curve).

Table 3. Dyssynchrony indexes: univariate logistic regression analysis for CRT response.

	Univariate Logistic Regression Analysis (Responder: ΔLVESV $\geq$ 15%)
	Odds Ratio [OR]; 95% Confidence Interval. ('p' Value)
Atrioventricular Dyssynchrony	
LVDFT/RR (Left Ventricular Diastolic Filling Time/RR time) (%)	0.963; 95% CI = 0.89–1.038 (p = 0.32)
LVDFT/RR < 40% (0/1)	0.5; 95% CI = 0.12–1.98 (p = 0.31)
Interventricular Dyssynchrony	
IVMD (Interventricular Mechanical Delay) (ms)	0.999; 95% CI = 0.98–1.02 (p = 0.99)
IVMD $\geq$ 40 ms (0/1)	1.07; 95% CI = 0.29–3.96 (p = 0.92)
Intraventricular Dyssynchrony	
Septal flash (0/1)	1.56; 95% CI = 0.34–7.17 (p = 0.56)
SPWMD (Septal to Posterior Wall Motion Delay) (ms)	0.999; 95% CI = 0.995–1.004 (p = 0.95)
4-chamber max intraventricular delay (ms)	0.99; 95% CI = 0.989–1.004 (p = 0.39)
Maximum Time Delay Technique (ms)	0.997; 95% CI = 0.99–1.003 (p = 0.29)
Maximal Opposing Wall Delay (ms)	0.996; 95% CI = 0.99–1.003 (p = 0.29)
Yu Index (ms)	0.993; 95% CI = 0.977–1.009 (p = 0.37)
Strain Pattern Analysis and RSPI	
General Classical Pattern (0/1)	1.95; 95% CI = 0.51–7.4 (p = 0.32)
RSPI (General Score)	1.26; 95% CI = 0.98–1.61 (p = 0.068)
RSPI $\geq$ 4 points	1.84; 95% CI = 0.42–8.06 (p = 0.41)
RSPI $\geq$ 7 points	12; 95% CI = 1.33–108.17 (p = 0.027)

Note: RSPI: Regional Strain Pattern Index.

4. Discussion

Numerous approaches have been proposed to quantify dyssynchrony and to improve patient's selection for CRT implantation [12,13]. In this study, we have presented our innovative proposal for the prediction of CRT response. We have introduced and verified the clinical use of RSPI. Our modified analysis of the contraction strain curve pattern was aimed at minimizing and overcoming the limitations of the previously employed echocardiographic indices of LV dyssynchrony.

RSPI is based on the assumption that dyssynchrony is a quantitative rather than qualitative process and RSPI reflects the severity of the disease. RSPI is expected to be effective also in a scarred myocardium. In the segments with an impaired contractility, the lack of a strain curve makes it impossible to define the strain pattern. However, in such a case, the features of intraventricular dyssynchrony may be present in other segments/views. Theoretically, this remaining portion of dyssynchrony in the viable segments may be revealed by RSPI and is believed to be a potential indicator for a positive response to CRT. Therefore, it is expected that a high RSPI score will identify responders even in case of patients with scarred segments and abnormal regional contractility.

Four important issues are listed below along with an explanation of why RSPI appears to be better than other methods for predicting the beneficial effects of CRT.

Firstly, it is a quantitative approach to dyssynchrony. Some of the classical, aforementioned parameters are based on rigid cut-off values or on the presence of specific signs such as a septal flash. We assumed that dyssynchrony (and the CRT response as well) is a "continuous" value and that it cannot be treated solely in terms of "presence" or "absence".

Secondly, it is a composite appraisal of dyssynchrony. The advantage of RSPI is that it takes into account dyssynchrony in 12 regions (three apical views with four segments in each view). Previous investigators have shown that the cumulative score of dyssynchrony increases the responsiveness to CRT [14,15]. In the classical parameters, the diminished contractility of one wall may lead to incorrect results. In RSPI, even in the case of impaired myocardial viability in one region, features of dyssynchrony may be present in the remaining regions. Therefore, the final RSPI could remain high, thus reflecting an existing dyssynchrony. Moreover, RSPI reflects changes during the entire cardiac cycle, not just in the ejection period.

Thirdly, the contractility. Patients without preserved contractility are unlikely to have a positive response to CRT. Abnormal contractility modifies the strain-derived pattern of LBBB [16]. Decreased contractility and scarring may predict a poor response to CRT regardless of the pathogenesis of cardiomyopathy [17,18]. Our innovative parameter indirectly assesses the contractility. The absence of contraction makes it impossible to assess the strain curves. Therefore, RSPI would not be scored in these regions (which actually means a "0" point).

Fourthly, the feasibility and simplicity. Many of the proposed dyssynchrony parameters require either specialized software or complex calculations [19]. To calculate RSPI, there is no need for extra tooling or to transfer the images to another system for the final processing of the results. RSPI calculation is possible ad hoc while performing a basic echocardiography examination.

Measurements of various dyssynchrony parameters were performed (Table 3). Among all of the indexes, only RSPI ≥ 7 points showed a significant relation with the CRT response in the univariate model (OR: 12; 95% CI 1.33–108.17; $p = 0.027$), whereas the general RSPI reached a borderline statistical significance (OR: 1.26; 95% CI 0.98–1.61; $p = 0.068$). Therefore, maybe the innovative quantitative methods based on strain analysis would be useful in improving the identification of CRT responders. Recently, Gorcsan et al. [20] proposed Systolic Stretch Index (SSI)—similar to our methodology based on strain analysis. SSI was strongly associated with favorable clinical outcomes including in the important patient subgroup with QRS width 120 to 149 ms or non-LBBB.

In our study, we intended to prove the usefulness of RSPI in case of all the patients who met the CRT criteria. Our group reflects the real-life, potential CRT recipients. In daily clinical practice, it is not only LBBB but also patients with non-LBBB and patients with CIED that undergo an up-grade procedure. Overall, the positive and negative predictive values of RSPI are quite modest but we must keep in mind that the study population was heterogeneous with different baseline conditions. Within the whole perspective, among the patients with different kinds of CRT indications, RSPI was positively verified with a specificity at satisfactory level of 92.3%.

The arguments presented in the discussion show that the evaluation of dyssynchrony is a composite, multifaceted problem. The Regional Strain Pattern Index is our new approach and has the potential to become a simple and practical tool for everyday use.

5. Limitations

Some limitations to our study should be addressed:

(1) It was a single center study. The study sample was small and quite heterogeneous (some patients had atrial fibrillation, while some had non-LBBB). Therefore, the predictive value of RSPI should be validated in a larger study with a more homogeneous population.
(2) The quality of the echocardiographic examination is crucial for image-based measurements of dyssynchrony. Suboptimal image quality may affect the results. From 71 consecutive patients qualified to enter into the study, finally six (8.5%) patients were excluded due to poor echocardiographic window.
(3) Strain pattern methodology relies on visual evaluation of the strain-derived curves. Therefore, during RSPI assessment, in some cases there may be discrepancies between observers.
(4) RSPI is a single parameter and reflects intraventricular dyssynchrony, whereas dyssynchrony and the response to CRT are multimodal ones. The selection of the most appropriate candidate for CRT might require a combined approach rather than a single parameter.
(5) The QRS duration criterion for entry into the study was 120 ms (according to the previous guidelines), whereas at present the cut-off value is 130 ms. However, no patient had a QRS shorter than 140 ms in our population.
(6) Post-implantation CRT optimization was not taken into consideration.

6. Conclusions

RSPI constitutes an innovative, valuable predictor for a CRT response. RSPI value of ≥ 7 points is an independent predictor of CRT response. RSPI appears to be better than the previously used dyssynchrony indexes for selecting patients for CRT and for efficiently identifying long-term responders.

Author Contributions: Conceptualization K.M.-S. and M.O.; methodology K.M.-S., W.O.; software W.W. and M.O.; validation K.M.-S., E.P.-G.; formal analysis W.W., A.B.-K.; investigation W.O., A.F., D.U.-S., W.K.; writing—original draft preparation M.O.; writing—review and editing, M.O.; visualization M.O.; supervision K.M.-S., A.F.; project administration A.F.; funding acquisition K.M.-S. All authors have read and agreed to the published version of the manuscript.

Funding: Grant for scientific research in the field of CRT efficacy funded by Medical University of Silesia.

Institutional Review Board Statement: The study was conducted according to the guidelines of the Declaration of Helsinki, and approved by Ethics Committee of Medical University of Silesia. Resolution with a positive opinion of Committee: Nr KNW/0022/KB1/123/13, dated 03.12.2013.

Informed Consent Statement: Informed consent was obtained from all subjects involved in the study.

Data Availability Statement: Not applicable.

Conflicts of Interest: The authors declare no conflict of interest.

References

1. Bristow, M.R.; Saxon, L.A.; Boehmer, J.; Krueger, S.; Kass, D.A.; De Marco, T.; Carson, P.; Dicarlo, L.; DeMets, D.; White, B.G.; et al. Cardiac-resynchronization therapy with or without an implantable defibrillator in advanced chronic heart failure. *N. Engl. J. Med.* **2004**, *350*, 2140–2150. [CrossRef] [PubMed]
2. Cleland, J.G.; Daubert, J.-C.; Erdmann, E.; Freemantle, N.; Gras, D.; Kappenberger, L.; Tavazzi, L. The effect of cardiac resynchronization on morbidity and mortality in heart failure. *N. Engl. J. Med.* **2005**, *352*, 1539–1549. [CrossRef] [PubMed]
3. Rossi, A.; Rossi, G.; Piacenti, M.; Startari, U.; Panchetti, L.; Morales, M.-A. The current role of cardiac resynchronization therapy in reducing mortality and hospitalization in heart failure patients: A meta-analysis from clinical trials. *Heart Vessel.* **2008**, *23*, 217–223. [CrossRef] [PubMed]
4. Cleland, J.G.; Daubert, J.-C.; Erdmann, E.; Freemantle, N.; Gras, D.; Kappenberger, L.; Tavazzi, L. Longer-term effects of cardiac resynchronization therapy on mortality in heart failure [the CArdiac REsynchronization-Heart Failure (CARE-HF) trial extension phase]. *Eur. Heart J.* **2006**, *27*, 1928–1932. [CrossRef] [PubMed]
5. Risum, N. Assessment of mechanical dyssynchrony in cardiac resynchronization therapy. *Dan. Med. J.* **2014**, *61*, B4981. [PubMed]
6. Parsai, C.; Bijnens, B.; Sutherland, G.R.; Baltabaeva, A.; Claus, P.; Marciniak, M.; Paul, V.; Scheffer, M.; Donal, E.; Derumeaux, G.; et al. Toward understanding response to cardiac resynchronization therapy: Left ventricular dyssynchrony is only one of multiple mechanisms. *Eur. Heart J.* **2009**, *30*, 940–949. [CrossRef] [PubMed]
7. Turner, M.; Bleasdale, R.; Vinereanu, D.; Mumford, C.E.; Paul, V.; Fraser, A.G.; Frenneaux, M.P. Electrical and mechanical components of dyssynchrony in heart failure patients with normal QRS duration and left bundle-branch block: Impact of left and biventricular pacing. *Circulation* **2004**, *109*, 2544–2549. [CrossRef] [PubMed]
8. To, A.C.Y.; Benatti, R.D.; Sato, K.; Grimm, R.A.; Thomas, J.D.; Wilkoff, B.L.; Agler, D.; Thamilarasan, M. Strain-time curve analysis by speckle tracking echocardiography in cardiac resynchronization therapy: Insight into the pathophysiology of responders vs. non-responders. *Cardiovasc. Ultrasound* **2016**, *14*, 14. [CrossRef] [PubMed]
9. Risum, N.; Jons, C.; Olsen, N.T.; Fritz-Hansen, T.; Bruun, N.E.; Hojgaard, M.V.; Valeur, N.; Kronborg, M.B.; Kisslo, J.; Sogaard, P. Simple regional strain pattern analysis to predict response to cardiac resynchronization therapy: Rationale, initial results, and advantages. *Am. Heart J.* **2012**, *163*, 697–704. [CrossRef] [PubMed]
10. Brignole, M.; Auricchio, A.; Baron-Esquivias, G.; Bordachar, P.; Boriani, G.; Breithardt, O.-A.; Cleland, J.G.F.; Deharo, J.-C.; Delgado, V.; Elliott, P.M.; et al. 2013 ESC Guidelines on cardiac pacing and cardiac resynchronization therapy: The Task Force on cardiac pacing and resynchronization therapy of the European Society of Cardiology (ESC). Developed in collaboration with the European Heart Rhythm Association. *Europace* **2013**, *15*, 1070–1118. [PubMed]
11. Prinzen, F.W.; Hunter, W.C.; Wyman, B.T.; McVeigh, E.R. Mapping of regional myocardial strain and work during ventricular pacing: Experimental study using magnetic resonance imaging tagging. *J. Am. Coll. Cardiol.* **1999**, *33*, 1735–1742. [CrossRef]
12. Yu, C.-M.; Fung, J.W.-H.; Zhang, Q.; Chan, C.K.; Chan, Y.-S.; Lin, H.; Kum, L.C.; Kong, S.-L.; Zhang, Y.; Sanderson, J.E.; et al. Tissue Doppler imaging is superior to strain rate imaging and postsystolic shortening on the prediction of reverse remodeling in both ischemic and nonischemic heart failure after cardiac resynchronization therapy. *Circulation* **2004**, *110*, 66–73. [CrossRef] [PubMed]
13. Suffoletto, M.S.; Dohi, K.; Cannesson, M.; Saba, S.; Gorcsan, J. Novel speckle-tracking radial strain from routine black-and-white echocardiographic images to quantify dyssynchrony and predict response to cardiac resynchronization therapy. *Circulation* **2006**, *113*, 960–968. [CrossRef] [PubMed]
14. Miyazaki, C.; Lin, G.; Powell, B.D.; Espinosa, R.E.; Bruce, C.J.; Miller, F.A.; Karon, B.L.; Rea, R.F.; Hayes, D.L.; Oh, J.K.; et al. Strain dyssynchrony index correlates with improvement in left ventricular volume after cardiac resynchronization therapy better than tissue velocity dyssynchrony indexes. *Circ. Cardiovasc. Imaging* **2008**, *1*, 14–22. [CrossRef] [PubMed]
15. Lim, P.; Donal, E.; Lafitte, S.; Derumeaux, G.; Habib, G.; Réant, P.; Thivolet, S.; Lellouche, N.; Grimm, R.A.; Gueret, P. Multicentre study using strain delay index for predicting response to cardiac resynchronization therapy (MUSIC study). *Eur. J. Heart Fail.* **2011**, *13*, 984–991. [CrossRef] [PubMed]
16. Leenders, G.E.; Lumens, J.; Cramer, M.J.; De Boeck, B.W.; Doevendans, P.A.; Delhaas, T.; Prinzen, F.W. Septal deformation patterns delineate mechanical dyssynchrony and regional differences in contractility: Analysis of patient data using a computer model. *Circ. Heart Fail.* **2012**, *5*, 87–96. [CrossRef] [PubMed]
17. Ahmed, W.; Samy, W.; Tayeh, O.; Behairy, N.; Abd El Fattah, A. Left ventricular scar impact on left ventricular synchronization parameters and outcomes of cardiac resynchronization therapy. *Int. J. Cardiol.* **2016**, *222*, 665–670. [CrossRef] [PubMed]
18. Morishima, I.; Okumura, K.; Tsuboi, H.; Morita, Y.; Takagi, K.; Yoshida, R.; Nagai, H.; Tomomatsu, T.; Ikai, Y.; Terada, K.; et al. Impact of basal inferolateral scar burden determined by automatic analysis of 99mTc-MIBI myocardial perfusion SPECT on the long-term prognosis of cardiac resynchronization therapy. *Europace* **2017**, *19*, 573–580. [CrossRef] [PubMed]
19. Werys, K.; Petryka-Mazurkiewicz, J.; Błaszczyk, Ł.; Misko, J.; Śpiewak, M.; Małek, Ł.A.; Miłosz-Wieczorek, B.; Marczak, M.; Kubik, A.; Dąbrowska, A.; et al. Cine dyscontractility index: A novel marker of mechanical dyssynchrony that predicts response to cardiac resynchronization therapy. *J. Magn. Reson. Imaging* **2016**, *44*, 1483–1492. [CrossRef] [PubMed]
20. Gorcsan, J.; Anderson, C.P.; Tayal, B.; Sugahara, M.; Walmsley, J.; Starling, R.C.; Lumens, J. Systolic Stretch Characterizes the Electromechanical Substrate Responsive to Cardiac Resynchronization Therapy. *JACC Cardiovasc. Imaging* **2019**, *12*, 1741–1752. [CrossRef] [PubMed]

MDPI
St. Alban-Anlage 66
4052 Basel
Switzerland
Tel. +41 61 683 77 34
Fax +41 61 302 89 18
www.mdpi.com

International Journal of Environmental Research and Public Health Editorial Office
E-mail: ijerph@mdpi.com
www.mdpi.com/journal/ijerph

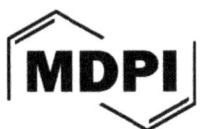

www.ingramcontent.com/pod-product-compliance
Lightning Source LLC
LaVergne TN
LVHW070557100526
838202LV00012B/486